ASSESSMENT and DOCUMENTATION:

Nursing Theories in Action

ANNITA B. WATSON, R.N., M.S.
Professor of Nursing
California State University
Sacramento, California

MARLENE G. MAYERS, R.N., M.S., F.A.A.N.
Assistant Administrator
Nursing Services
Rosecliff Community Hospital
Rosecliff, California

Preface

The idea for this text originated with the students and staff nurses who have shared with us their struggles to gather, organize, and document client information. We have read innumerable books on the subjects of assessment and documentation, each presenting a piece of the total picture. Some references discuss conceptual frameworks and theories, others detail specific charting methods, still others explain nursing audit and imply the necessity for change in charting practices. We have not found one reference based on a conceptual framework that is comprehensive in content and still practical in its approach. This book represents our attempt to provide such a textbook for practitioners of nursing.

In this book, assessment and documentation is presented in such a way that the content becomes meaningful and workable in both educational and service settings. We show, explain, and apply assessment guides and documentation methods to a variety of client situations. Each chapter sets forth practical approaches for the implementation of its content. We have provided the reader with detailed examples of "how to" assess and document.

The book is divided into five chapters. The first chapter establishes the conceptual framework for the entire book. It defines assessment and documentation and answers the question: "How can we know why we do what we do?" The answer lies in a conceptual framework: its constructs, concepts, and theories. How to make a theory work for the real world of nursing practice is explained and demonstrated.

Chapter 2 focuses on assessment in action by explaining how to observe, question, inspect, and deduce. Various data collection methods are illustrated, incorporating retrieval of both expected and unexpected data. The chapter explains each phase of the assessment process, from data collection through nursing diagnosis.

Chapter 3 presents documentation as a process of assembling, coding, and disseminating information according to the guidelines established by the conceptual framework. Three major methods are illustrated in detail, by means of case studies.

Integration of theories, algorithms, assessment, and documentation are discussed in chapter 4. Many client situations illustrate assessment algorithms. Four major case studies demonstrate comprehensive application of theory-based assessment and documentation.

The final chapter analyzes existing models for assessment and documentation and shows how to adapt them to reflect theories in use, and ways to revise them to be consistent with suitable theories.

In writing this book, we became more than ever aware of the importance of the conceptual framework. Several attempts to explain and illustrate assessment were rejected before we accepted the fact that a theoretical base for practice, as exemplified in this book, is necessary. The conceptual framework we developed enabled us to define our terms, to converse with one another, and to defend our rationale. We were delighted, of course, with our enhanced abilities in communication, and with the discovery that we could, in fact, work inductively and deductively in testing theories. Of special importance to us was the discovery that this book's content became valuable to us both, with each of us operating in a different setting — education and service.

It is important that, as authors, we point out that our use of constructs, concepts, and theories for the formulation of assessment guides is arbitrary, and is based on our personal conceptions, experiences, and collaboration. Others, using the same constructs, concepts, and theories, may arrive at different interpretations which can be equally valid. Our framework serves as a tool, enabling us to illustrate a process. This framework was developed because of recognition that nursing assessment must be based on a common interpretation of nursing as a profession, of the nursing client, and of the knowledge basic to good nursing performance. A conceptual framework already developed might have been used. Instead, it was decided to use a new framework in order to avoid a presumptuous interpretation of someone else's work. Further, we recognized the need to work through the conceptual process of framework development in order to achieve an acceptable frame of reference for this writing. It is, however, probable that the conceptual framework here is not significantly different from many others, primarily because of similar definitions accepted. In no way do we suggest to our readers that "our" way is "the" way to interpret theories within a conceptual framework.

A complete conceptual framework includes more detail than we have presented. We have arbitrarily selected those portions that proved useful to us as we illustrated specific points within this book. We have touched briefly on other details that are important to include in a comprehensive, operational, conceptual framework.

We express sincere appreciation to the many students, nursing staff, and colleagues who helped test our ideas and hunches. We appreciate both their enthusiasm and their careful criticisms as our work progressed. We especially acknowledge Jean Altman and Marilyn Kempton for their constant human conceptual and technical help.

Authors' Note

We recognize that both men and women are nurses; however, to avoid redundancy, we use the pronoun "she" when referring to nurses. We also have tended to use the term "client" rather than "patient" when referring to consumers of health care.

Contents

To Our Families

1

A Framework for Assessment and Documentation

How often has the nurse asked herself: Why do I ask the questions I do? Why do I make certain physical inspections and not others? Why do I make certain observations and record them, or why do I make other observations and ignore them? How much do biases, traditions or roles play a part in what I choose to ask, or to observe, or to chart? How many observations and decisions rest upon a rationale or theory that can be defined or supported? All such questions relate to establishing a framework for assessment and documentation.

The answers to these questions come from many sources and efforts, one of which is the focus of this book. These issues are examined from the standpoint of conceptual frameworks and theories as a basis for defining what is to be assessed and what is to be clearly documented. It has been claimed that nursing, as taught and practiced today, is primarily intuitive.[1] There are other claims that the answers to the dilemma posed by these questions lie in theory-based practice.

Theory here is based on the belief that through systematic assessment and documentation the theoretical roots of nursing can be clarified, developed, articulated, and evaluated. This book includes several new approaches to systematic assessment and documentation. To accomplish the purpose of this text, a conceptual framework equally applicable to the educational or service setting has been developed. Specific theories have been arbitrarily selected to interpret the client of nursing and the practice of nursing. These theories have provided the basis for a step-by-step process whereby data-gathering guides can be formulated. Utilization of these assessment guides results in formulation of theory-based nursing diagnoses. These diagnoses relate directly to a series of health standards that are in turn derived from theories.

Documentation of this type of assessment provides a frame of reference for practice in any given situation. It offers justification for decisions. It has been found that a systematic approach to documentation gives a foundation for professional credibility. This has fostered communication, dialogue, and constructive criticism among nurses, between nurses and clients, and between nursing and other disciplines. Theory helps the nurse to justify her own actions. Rather than say: "I did it because it seemed best," she can say: "I did it because of my interpretation of the situation relative to a specific theory or theories." When nursing can specifically justify its decisions and actions, it fulfills its contract with society.

Society itself is demanding greater accountability from all the professions. It is asking clear processes of internal review and self-regulation. It is also imposing external methods of control through a myriad of regulations. Consumers are asking many questions: "Why have health-care costs soared?" "What am I getting for my health-care dollar?" "Who is accountable for my care?" "Is health care consistent with client values, or only with those of the professionals?" The advent of consumer rights has accelerated the need for clear lines of accountability. As clients have exerted their rights through pressure groups, legal actions, and legislation, it has become crystal clear to nurses that practice by intuition or by the medical model is insufficient.

In spite of nursing's long history of concern for and care for people, confusion still exists.[2,3] Nurses and consumers alike are wondering who the nurse is and what unique function the nurse fulfills. If nurses are to be responsible and accountable to society, to colleagues, and to clients, they must be able to define and articulate their body of knowledge. Their social mandate cannot be met unless they can clearly explain what they do and how and why they do it. They must be practitioners who are "able to use the scientific method for the analysis and resolution of health care problems...observations must be recorded routinely and systematically, and generalizing questions must be asked which derive from these clinical data."[2] A basis for nursing practice must be developed through research. This can be done either formally or informally, and either inductively or deductively.[4] Inductive research scrutinizes nursing practice as it exists, in an attempt to formulate hunches or hypotheses that can be tested and that will ultimately lead to a theory of nursing science. Or, a current body of knowledge can be organized through a conceptual framework, generally accepted theories selected and applied to nursing, then tested for validity, thereby producing deductive nursing theory.

So, whether inductive or deductive reasoning is used in routine day-to-day practice, the careful documentation of thought, action, and outcome preserves the intellectual basis of nursing for further study.

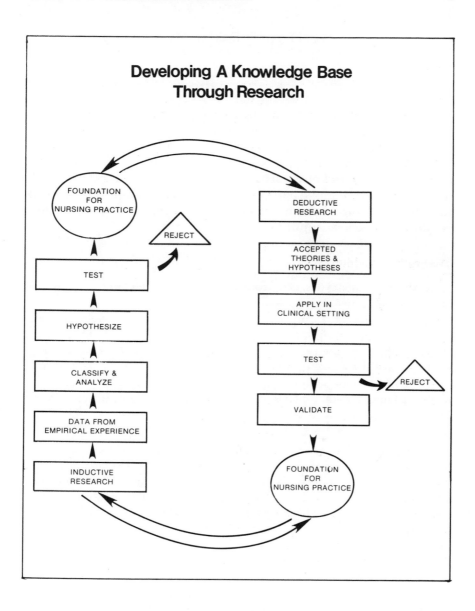

Developing A Knowledge Base Through Research

ASSESSMENT AND DOCUMENTATION

Assessment

Within the context of this book, assessment is defined as a systematic collection of data for the purpose·of diagnosing a client's health status. This definition requires that theory-based criteria and standards be used as a basis for interviewing, inspecting, observing, analyzing, interpreting, and judging. The end phase of assessment is a nursing diagnosis. Assessment refers to an initial diagnosis as well as to a dynamic ongoing confirmation or change of diagnosis. This definition encompasses theoretical validity and practical application.

Theoretical Validity

All the assessment cues, questions, inspection guides, and standards for decisions developed here are systematically derived from a cluster of theories relating to a concept. These assessment guides represent the authors' interpretation of the theories, and have not been field-tested for construct validity or reliability. Such testing is needed and is therefore part of the task of deductive research in nursing. The reader is encouraged to focus attention on the systematic processes depicted in the text, and is cautioned not to become distracted by the authors' arbitrary interpretations of theories.

Practical Application

The systematic assessment processes outlined in the text are designed to assist the nurse to collect, organize, and analyze data quickly. Steps and rules for decision-making are presented and illustrated in actual client-care situations. A data-gathering format rooted in theory has been developed here; it guides the nurse quickly and comprehensively through all the phases of the assessment process.

Documentation

In this text documentation is defined as the act of assembling, coding, and disseminating information in written form. It must provide factual or substantial support for statements made, or for hypotheses proposed. Thus, documentation preserves the facts and substantial elements of the nursing process and the clients' responses, for constant, careful scrutiny. This definition assumes formalized methods of assembling data with rules for use.

Current methods of documentation are explained and illustrated. Client-care situations are used to illustrate documentation on the nursing history, the chart, and the care plan. Other documentation forms, such as referral forms and flow sheets, are also illustrated.

Although assessment and documentation can occur on many levels, the focus here is the assessment and documentation of the client by the nurse. A variety of client-care settings are used to illustrate these processes.

CONCEPTUAL FRAMEWORK

What is a conceptual framework?How can it help nursing practice? Consider what would happen if a builder proceeded to construct a house without a blueprint. Or, think about how a symphony would sound if all 60 musicians attempted to play Mozart, each from his own perception of how it should sound. What would happen if a group of nurses attempted to care for a client without commonly understood knowledge and guidelines for practice? Each nurse would "do her own thing," in her own way, according to her own rationale and her own interpretation of the situation. Imagine what happens to the client when each of 20 nurses performs according to her individual perception of the situation.

A builder is expected to follow an architect's plan. That plan is expected to reflect the people who will live in the house, their lifestyle, their preferences for texture and color, and their economic resources. In the same way, one prefers to hear Mozart played from a single score. And a client undoubtedly prefers nurses with commonly understood perceptions about nursing and about the persons for whom they are caring. In academic and professional disciplines the "blueprint" or the musical "score" is referred to as a conceptual framework.

> A conceptual framework is a description of a group's ideas about the world for which it is responsible. This description defines each part of that world and explains how each part fits together and functions to create a "whole," thereby enabling the group to predict the results of its actions.

A conceptual framework is a set of statements describing one's ideas or notions about a desired or predicted reality, world, or universe, which one wishes or needs to control. In this definition, "world" means the total entity for which the nurse is responsible. It can be a total nursing curriculum, a total nursing-service program, a total health agency, or one total service within a larger agency. To visualize a universe in order to formulate a conceptual framework, one needs to identify and define the component parts, their functions, the characteristics of each part, as well as the way in which these parts interrelate to one another and to the total universe.

A conceptual framework implies or prescribes specific expectations and outcomes of the universe and its parts. It guides the decisions of those who are using it so that their intentions can be realized. A conceptual framework reflects a combination of beliefs, purposes, empirical experience, and scientific research. Those who would advance the professional practice of nursing must have a sound basis, a conceptual framework, on which to build their view of their professional practice. That framework must be constructed from validated empirical knowledge and from the discovery of new information acquired through the efforts of nurse-scientists, scholars, and practitioners.

To clarify the definition and interpretation of a conceptual framework, the analogy of the architect as he plans his building can again the considered. The building is the universe, the reality he wishes to control. His expectation is that he will prepare plans and specifications to result in the completion of a structure now seen only in his mind. To bring his idealized building into reality, he must be able to transcribe to paper the information which will allow others to know what materials to use and how to use them. But he must also have sufficient knowledge to recognize which materials are suitable for his purposes, which will be strong enough or flexible enough to sustain weight, and which will meet a variety of other requirements.

Using such knowledge, he draws a plan for his building, noting on the blueprint all necessary information. He may also write detailed specifications, listing the materials to be used and the ways in which they are to be employed. By so doing, he has converted the mental picture of the building he wants to construct into steel, concrete, wood, and stone.

A conceptual framework for a nursing program or service must work in much the same way. Its designers must decide what it is they want to achieve. They must know the ingredients that make such a conception possible. They must also know how to employ the necessary methods to turn their knowledge into reality. In essence, the conceptual framework may be viewed as a blueprint for the program.

Such a framework serves as a guide for making program decisions and for systematically evaluating those decisions in practice. It gives perspective and a sense of relationship to all the factors involved in the development of nursing practice. By defining the various parts and showing how they relate to one another, the conceptual framework allows a view of the larger whole and makes possible the development of criteria for the assessment, documentation, and evaluation of client status, nursing performance, and program evaluation.

A Conceptual Framework for Assessment and Documentation

The conceptual framework developed here is equally functional for a nursing-education curriculum or for a nursing-service program. The framework represents values, biases, and beliefs. It is eclectic in nature, using theories from many disciplines. It is an example of a comprehensive framework.

Constructs, Concepts, Theories

Since the conceptual framework describes a universe, its parts, and their relationships, it must be organized in some way that vividly depicts these parts and their relationships. Depending upon one's "universe," the organizing parts will vary. In nursing, many educational programs identify four major constructs as the organizers for their conceptual framework. These four constructs are *Man, Society, Health,* and *Nursing.*[5] These same constructs are useful organizers for conceptual frameworks in nursing-service programs.[6,7,8,9,10,11,12] Many nursing faculty and staff experience confusion and frustration when confronted with need to develop a conceptual framework. Organizers or constructs serve as guides for formulating a set of descriptive statements representative of the beliefs of a faculty or of a nursing-service staff. These four constructs seem to encompass all aspects of nursing. An education or service program, however, is not limited to these four constructs.

Other professional disciplines have their own conceptual frameworks and constructs which may resemble those for nursing, or which may vary widely. The field of social work may easily use the same four constructs. By contrast, the discipline of accounting undoubtedly has different major ocnstructs for its educational programs and fields of practice.

Constructs

A construct is a classification of ideas. It is a label that represents many ideas or experiences that have similar characteristics. Constructs are general organizers of large amounts of information.

> A construct is a general label that classifies large amounts of information.

Labeling or organizing enables the individual to recall information. It also enables him to further subdivide and categorize ideas that fall under that broad label. For example, *food* can be considered a construct referring to many kinds of edible products. Similarity lies in the fact that when one hears the label *food*, one thinks of eating rather than of putting on clothing. Nursing can be considered a construct. It conjures up ideas different from those of medicine 0r law. Since constructs are broad and abstract, vulnerable to multiple interpretations, it is necessary for a group to further define its interpretation of the construct through more specific labels called *concepts*.

Concepts

A concept is also a label describing clusters of ideas and experiences which have things in common. Concepts are less general than constructs. What they really do is interpret the construct. For example, the construct *food* may conjure up such concepts as American, Chinese, French, Italian, or other cuisines. Or it may conjure a very different set of ideas — for example, low-calorie, low-cholesterol, high-protein, or high-fiber foods. The same analogy can be made of nursing. The construct itself leads to many different sets of interpretations: technical, professional, vocational, primary, team, and so forth. It is, therefore, necessary to use concepts to define and describe constructs.

> A concept is a label which describes clusters of ideas and experiences which have characteristics in common.

The terms *construct* and *concept* are not consistently used the same way in the literature. Many references do not use the term *construct* at all, mentioning only the terms *concepts*, and *sub-concepts* to describe their labels. Others refer to constructs as "high-level concepts."[13,14] The latter interpretation is consistent with the way the terms are used in this text. The terms *Man, Society, Health,* and *Nursing* are identified here as high-level concepts or constructs.

The following diagram interprets the parallel use of the terms *construct* and *concept*.

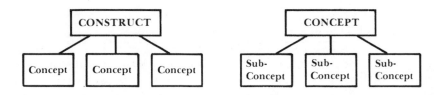

In either case, the terms *concept* and *sub-concept* definitively describe a group's interpretation of the higher-level concept or construct. One group can define man (construct) as a bio-psycho-social spiritual being (concept). Another group can define man (construct) as a biological organism governed by physiological needs (concept). For the purposes of this text, a concept is a label for a set of things with something in common.[15] It is a generalized idea or organization of a group of related phenomena that communicates an image or mental picture. It classifies experiences that have similar properties. Concepts are significant and important in and of themselves. In addition, concepts are the ideas out of which theories are built.[16] Concepts can also be basic elements in the structure of a theory.[17]

Theories

A theory is a statement of a scientifically acceptable relationship between two or more phenomena or factors which describes, explains, and predicts consequences and results.[16,18] To be useful, a theory must contain definitions of its terms, the assumptions upon which it rests, and its hypotheses.[19] A theory is a way of organizing information to make it understandable and practical.

> A theory is a statement of a relationship between two or more variables which describes, explains, or predicts.

Since human beings have a limited capacity to observe and recall, they are simply not able to perceive everything about them in totality. The world is too complex. Theories, then, are used by people to limit the observable world in order to help them be selective. Theories do not represent a totality. To understand a theory, one must think in terms of definitions, assumptions, and hypotheses.

Definitions—Definitions clearly describe terms so that all who read or use them will have the same frame of reference. For instance, the word "nurse" may have many definitions. A specific theory about a specific kind of nurse will clearly describe the meaning of nurse for that theory.

Assumptions—Assumptions describe the conditions under which the theory holds—what must be accepted as given in order to make that theory work. For example, a specific theory about a nurse may rest on the assumption that the nurse is working in a primary-care setting, or that a nurse can function independently in a collegial role. In essence then, one can not use a theory with these assumptions under any other conditions.

Hypotheses—Hypotheses are working guesses about how things behave and about the relationships between things in the real world. They must relate to the assumptions and to the terms defined in the theory. An hypothesis relative to the primary nurse may be this: *a primary nurse produces better care at lower cost than does another type of nurse.* The resulting theory, combining definitions, assumptions, and hypotheses may be: *a primary nurse is one who provides comprehensive care to a caseload of clients on a 24-hour basis. This nurse has the authority to make all nursing decisions for her clients. And because of her authority, knowledge, expertise, and freedom from hierarchical restraints she will provide comprehensive, quality care at a lower cost than if she were functioning in a team-concept situation.* The examples are not intended to be representative of a complete theory.

In summary, a conceptual framework is made up of constructs, concepts, and theories. These three components organize the intellectual basis for assessment and documentation. They reflect descending orders of abstraction, or increasing levels of specificity.

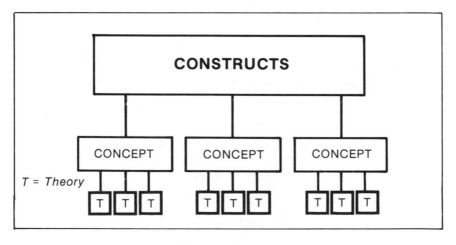

An Open Systems
Conceptual Framework

For the purposes of this text four constructs are being used: *Man, Environment, Health,* and *Nursing.* Each construct is clarified through concepts and theories. The concepts and theories represent the authors' meaning of the four constructs. An open-systems approach is used as a theme for the entire framework.

Figure 1.1 shows how these constructs and concepts are labeled. Looking only at the constructs, the arrows and the equation symbolize the reciprocal interaction of man and his environment to produce a state of health. The construct *nursing* is included as it interacts with the other three constructs.

CONSTRUCTS	MAN	ENVIRONMENT	HEALTH	NURSING
CONCEPTS	Systems:	Systems:	Energy	Functions:
	Physiological Psychological	Economic		Human
	Cognitive/ Intellectual	Physical		Conceptual
	Sensory/ Perceptive	Mobile		Technical
	Interactive/ Affiliative	Social/ Cultural		
	Mobile			

Figure 1.1
Conceptual Framework: An Open Systems Model

Concepts of Man

To define man, six concepts that represent an open-systems approach and that together interpret man as a holistic being have been selected. The six concepts (systems) are

- Physiological
- Psychological
- Cognitive
- Sensory/Perceptive
- Interactive/Affiliative
- Mobile

Man is a whole being consisting of millions of parts, in the form of cells, organs, and body systems. The body is inseparable from the psyche, and from man's interactions with the environment. What happens in any one of these parts affects the whole.

> Wholeness implies that the individual functions as a complete, well-integrated whole. All the various activities of the several parts of Man seem directed to central ends; thus, there is cooperation and unified action of the organism as a whole...[20]

> Man strives to be alert, to grow, to develop, and to perform the acts of daily living with interest, enjoyment, and satisfaction.[21]

> Thus, Man is viewed as an open system...interacting with his environment in a dynamic, continuous interchange...[22]

Concepts of Environment

Several concepts, or systems, are chosen to interpret the construct *environment*. They are:

- Economic
- Physical
- Mobile
- Demographic
- Social/Cultural

The environment is all those systems that produce stimuli or stressors affecting changes in man. Environment and Man are reciprocal systems in which molding and being molded are taking place simultaneously. Environmental and human fields are continuously repatterned. With each repatterning, subsequent interaction is revised and a new pattern is formed.[23]

Concept of Health

One concept, *energy*, is used to interpret health. Man's health is a dynamic, changing phenomenon, dependent upon the amount of energy available to him to carry out life's activities in a satisfactory way. Health is that composition of human and environmental factors that produces the greatest possible integrity for both. Health is the optimal combined mix of needs satisfied.[24] Energy serves as a catalyst for achieving this combined mix. Energy is not unlimited; it must be constantly replenished. Each system, man and environment, is both a consumer and a provider of energy. A state of health for both man and the environment occurs when there is a balance between energy supply and demand. Energy supply and demand arise from constant adjustments in an energy-conserving—energy-releasing equation. Man and environment strive to maintain a state of health by reciprocally adapting to stress in order to achieve a balance between the supply of and the demand for energy. This reciprocal adaptation produces changes in one, several, or all the systems.[25]

$$\text{MAN} \rightleftharpoons \text{ENVIRONMENT} = \text{HEALTH}$$

Concepts of Nursing

Nursing is interpreted through three concepts: human, conceptual, and technical functions. Each function requires both art and science. Nursing is designed to "promote symphonic interaction between Man and Environment, to strengthen the coherence and integrity of the human field, and to direct and redirect patterning of the human and environmental fields for realization of maximum health potential."[23]

Nursing as a human function is the "ability and judgment in working with and through people, involving an understanding of motivation, and an application of effective leadership skills."[26] It is "caring for the whole individual and his relation to his environment.... Caring means giving serious attention to someone, yet avoiding intrusion."[27] This humanistic approach is based on certain beliefs about man: he achieves uniqueness through interpersonal contact; he is aware of himself and his existence; he is capable of making choices which guide his own behavior.

Nursing as a conceptual function is that ability to understand the complexities of society, of one's organization, of one's own set of responsibilities and to function according to their objectives rather than upon only immediate or personal needs and goals. Conceptual functions are processes of forming or understanding ideas, abstractions, and symbols. These processes are generally seen as aiding a practitioner in focusing systematically on relevant facts and variables, in explaining basic causes, and in formulating predictions about probable outcomes.[28]

Nursing as a technical function is the ability to apply knowledge and to use specific skills to implement the activities of client-centered care. These activities encompass both direct and indirect elements of care. Application of knowledge occurs at various levels, in a variety of settings, and is designed to facilitate a positive, reciprocal interaction between man and his environment. These skills vary according to diverse settings and are performed in both structured and unstructured situations, with or without fixed expectations, guidelines, or regulations. Expertise is required in areas of technology, administration, education, and research. The degree and sophistication of expertise will differ according to roles and performance expectations.

The beliefs represented in these statements influence the selection of theories used in this conceptual framework.

THEORIES OF MAN, ENVIRONMENT, HEALTH, AND NURSING

Numerous theories are included in this conceptual framework. They are specifically selected for their consistency with the overriding "open-systems" theme, and with the authors' philosophy. Because of this open-systems theme, many of these theories overlap in their explanation of man's behavior, and many of them are holistic enough in their explanations that arbitrary decisions have been made as to which of man's systems they best interpret. This overlapping phenomenon is likely to occur in any conceptual framework if man is approached as a holistic being who interacts with his environment to achieve a state of health with a satisfactory level of energy. Fig. 1.2 outlines the theories selected for each of the concepts related to man, environment, health, and nursing.

THEORIES IN ACTION

Moment by moment in his daily life, the individual theorizes about something, whether he realizes it or not. Many lives are fashioned on the theory that going to work results in personal satisfaction and economic rewards that are worth the effort. Other people offer quite a different theory of personal satisfaction and economic reward, and therefore fashion their lives differently. Another prevalent theory in Western culture is that without the basic unit of society, the family, society would disintegrate. Most nurses in everyday practice focus on meeting acute physical needs before meeting learning or emotional needs. Whether they realize it or not, this type of priority is consistent with such a theory as Maslow's Hierarchy of Needs, which describes progressive levels of need fulfillment.[29]

Almost all the actions the nurse takes are really based upon some theory that allows her to predict the consequences or outcomes of her actions. She can usually explain the rationale for her actions and often refers to some theory such as "Maslow's Hierarchy of Needs" or "the process of communication." What she usually does not do, however, is to identify the rationale for action as theories. In fact, she may first tend to react with annoyance when asked to identify a theory or theorist. She wonders: Does it

Figure 1.2

Open-Systems Model: Constructs, Concepts, and Theories

MAN	⇄	ENVIRONMENT	⇌	HEALTH	NURSING
CONCEPTS AND THEORIES SYSTEMS: PHYSIOLOGICAL Reciprocal Adaptation Stress Growth and Development PSYCHOLOGICAL Need Motivation Growth and Development COGNITIVE/INTELLECTUAL Learning Stress SENSORY/PERCEPTIVE Perception Growth and Development INTERACTIVE/AFFILIATIVE Interpersonal Communication Group Role Cultural MOBILE Spatial Relations		CONCEPTS AND THEORIES SYSTEMS: ECONOMIC Supply and Demand PHYSICAL Systems — Ecology Air Pollution Water Pollution Noise Pollution Temperature/Humidity/ Light Alterations Radiation Exposure Chemical, Microbial, and Safety Hazards MOBILE Cultural Spatial Relations DEMOGRAPHIC Density SOCIAL/CULTURAL Ethnocentricity Organization Reciprocal Adaptation Interpersonal Communication Group/Role Intimacy Cultural		CONCEPTS AND THEORIES ENERGY Free Energy Energy Fields	CONCEPTS AND THEORIES FUNCTIONS: HUMAN Affective Development Humanistic Helping Systems Change Leadership Authority Power Influence Conflict Human Relations CONCEPTUAL Cognitive Development Theory Development Decision TECHNICAL Psychomotor Development Administration Education Research

make me sound snobbish? Does it really help me or my clients? Is there really any practical value, or is it a form of intellectual elitism?

However, the annoyance is replaced with a feeling of satisfaction when two colleagues can discuss a client situation from the same theoretical frame of reference. If a client is having a "communication problem," nurses may analyze the situation in terms of the process of communication as outlined by Ruesch,[30] or they may analyze the situation according to metacommunication theory as defined by Lewis.[31] When colleagues know both theories—definitions, assumptions, and hypotheses—they can consult with each other with clear understanding and expectations for both themselves and the clients. Theoretical frames of reference provide defenses for analyses and decisions, and furnish bases for criticizing or reviewing analyses, decisions, and actions. Without a theory, there is a tendency to practice by rote, by tradition, and by "the seat of the pants," hoping that perhaps there may later come an understanding of what was done, and why.

Theories, however, may or may not be sound. As good as they are, theories may represent an oversimplification of reality, may be outdated as reality changes, or may have been unsound to begin with. Both Maslow[29] and Erickson[32] are good cases in point. Their theories are widely used in nursing and other disciplines; however, many scholars argue that though the theories seem logical, they have been accepted without rigorous scientific testing. Thus, in putting theories into use, nurses are continuously testing them, modifying them, validating them, or discarding them. The ultimate benefit of using specific theory as a basis for action lies in its assistance in building and refining a body of knowledge.

How to Make a Theory Useful for Assessment

A theory helps one to focus. The focus lies in theory's major or main terms and definitions. The nurse can look at a theory and extract and list these terms. The list then establishes the parameters or limits for her attention. This list gives her the major criteria about which she needs information.

> A criterion is a value-free term which labels some element of a theory.

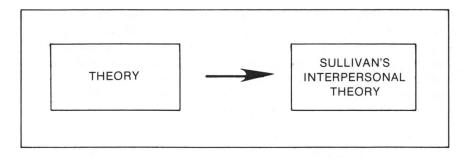

The nurse can now take a theory and abstract the terms, definitions, and criteria. Harry Stack Sullivan's interpersonal theory[33,34,35] is interesting. It applies to nursing and it lends itself well to extraction of terms.

Sullivan's theory states that everyone's goal in interpersonal situations is to feel approval and prestige and to avoid anxiety. People's interactive behavior, then, is designed to reduce tension and to enhance their own feelings of security. Furthermore, a person's feelings of anxiety or security are significantly influenced by past interactions with significant other people. Sullivan hypothesizes that:

- Tension reduction and security combine to become the major behavior goals of any individual
- To feel secure, an individual requires feelings of approval and prestige
- Perception of approval and prestige are the result of past and present experiences with significant others
- Past relationships influence perceptions of present relationships
- A person's own concept or self-dynamism organizes his behavior and is a result of past and present experiences with significant others
- Behavior, emotions, and needs originate from the interaction of one individual with another
- Anxiety is the chief disruptive force in interpersonal relationships
- Insecurity in interpersonal relationships produces anxiety
- A person will interact or not interact to reduce anxiety

This is a condensed version of Sullivan's theory and does not necessarily reflect the theory in its entirety. Scanning this condensed version, six major terms, criteria, that appear to be crucial elements are identified:

1. feelings of approval
2. feelings of prestige
3. anxiety, tension
4. self-dynamism, self-concept
5. interpersonal security

6. perceptions of past and present relationships or interactions

It should be noted that the criteria* are value-free labels of the important elements of the theory.[36] They are indications for assessing one's level of health. Since they are value-free, they do not in themselves tell how to make a judgment about one's level of interpersonal health. They do, however, suggest topics about which to gather information so that ultimately the nurse can decide how healthy an individual is.

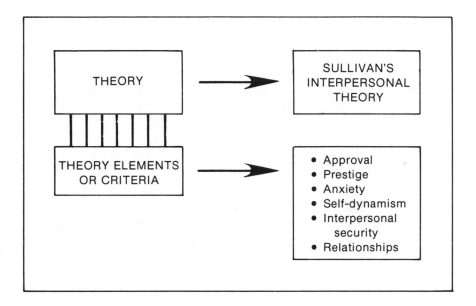

How to Assign a Value to a Criterion

To decide ultimately what a person's level of interpersonal health is, a standard is required.

> A standard is the desired and achievable level of performance relative to a criterion against which actual performance is compared.[36]

---

*This definition of criteria is different from the same term commonly referred to in quality-assurance literature where criteria often assume values.

A standard requires that a value be assigned to a criterion. The question is: how can it be known what value to assign? There are basically three ways of arriving at a value:

1. **Group norms:**[36,37,38] If enough is known about a specific group or population relative to the criterion, it is possible to assign a value that reflects the frequency distribution of the value among this population. For example, enough people have been weighed and measured for height to determine a normal weight for a given age and sex. By the same token, enough oral temperatures have been taken to determine that the normal oral temperature for an adult is 98.6°F. Thus, many clinical standards have already been mathematically established and are used in the nurse's daily practice. These standards represent group norms.

2. **Experts' opinions:**[39] In many cases not enough is known about a population and its normal distributions to arrive at a mathematical value. However, certain experts know much about particular levels of skills or competencies. For example, expert coronary-care nurses can predict that if a patient is progressing well, he will be demonstrating certain behavior by a certain time. The majority of standard-care plans and audit criteria represent experts' opinions and have not been statistically studied.

3. **Individual expectations:**[37,40,41] When group norms and experts' opinions are not known or are not judged desirable or appropriate, values are determined by an individual's decisions relative to the criterion. A personal value judgement is made.

These three ways of arriving at values (standards) may be used alone or in combination, depending upon one's purpose and knowledge of a situation. In the case of Sullivan's interpersonal theory, for example, the authors here designated themselves as experts. They reviewed and interpreted Sullivan's theory to formulate a standard: *The presence of feelings of security in the most important interpersonal relationships.* This represents "experts' opinions" which can be used as a standard to measure or judge an individual's interpersonal health. All health standards illustrated in this book are derived from the concept of energy. Values are assigned relative to theories of free energy[42] and energy fields.[23] Optimal health is achieved when man possesses enough energy to accomplish those things he desires to do. Less optimal health exists when there is only enough energy for man to do what he must. A minimal state of health exists when energy is limited to maintaining physiological survival. Man and environment are reciprocal energy fields striving to maintain an optimal balance.

Methods of Measurement
and Data Collection

In order to judge whether or not a client meets a health standard, some

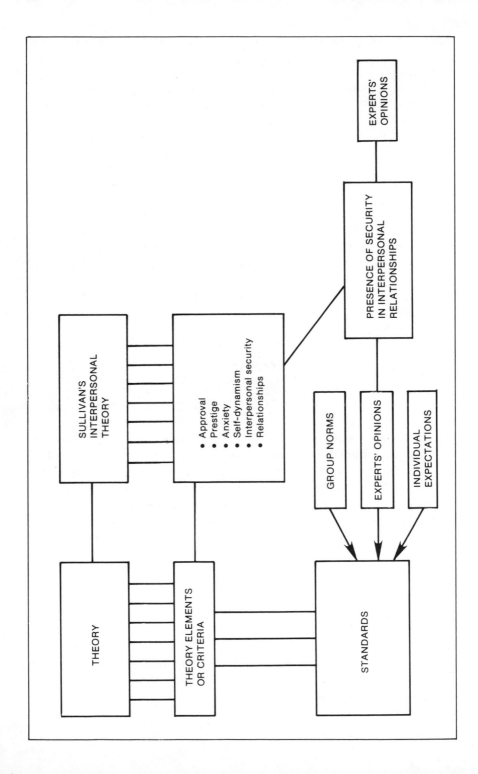

method of measurement must be used. In some cases it is either impractical or scientifically premature to have, or even to hope for, a fine testing measurement. For example, for Sullivan's theory there is no pure standardized test that relates specifically to the measurement of interpersonal security. Thus, less precise theory-related questions and observations must suffice. However, many physiological theories have well-developed testing methods and instruments: the thermometer, the electrocardiogram, the blood-chemistry panel, and others. Obviously, nurses will use a spectrum of measurement methods to gather data and make judgments. Methods of measurement are as precise as the mechanisms by which values are assigned to criteria. When group mathematical norms are well-known, precise measurement tests are likely to be available. When experts' opinions are used to set standards, experts also use their best judgment to design questions or observation cues. And in the case of individual situations, personal subjective judgments are relied upon for measurement.

The authors here also acted as experts in formulating for Sullivan's interpersonal theory a set of assessment (measurement) questions:

1. How do you feel about what is happening to you?
2. Who, if anyone, can help you or be supportive of you at this time?
3. How much control do you feel over what is happening to you?
4. Has anything like this ever happened before?
5. Who are the most important people in your life?
6. How comfortable or uncomfortable do you feel with these people?

In summary, the best method of measurement available is used to test (assess or determine) how well an individual or client compares to a standard. Decisions are easy when group-norm information is available. One score is simply compared with another. Expert practitioners make judgments about the meaning of the data gathered when expertly designed measurement tools are used. The same holds true when comparing data with individual decisions. Either the nurse or the client may well be qualified to make the value judgment regarding actual performance.

Judgments, Hypotheses, Diagnoses

The three terms—judgments, hypotheses, and diagnoses—can be used interchangeably. They are all testable conclusions derived from a systematic collection of data. If, after gathering data, the nurse judges that an individual's interpersonal health status meets or does not meet the standard, she has made a nursing diagnosis. This hypothesis will be tested as she implements a plan of action based upon her conclusions. This, in effect, tests the theory with which she began.

The entire process described here shows how, in making a nursing diagnosis, theories in action help nurses to focus their attention on the most relevant issues.

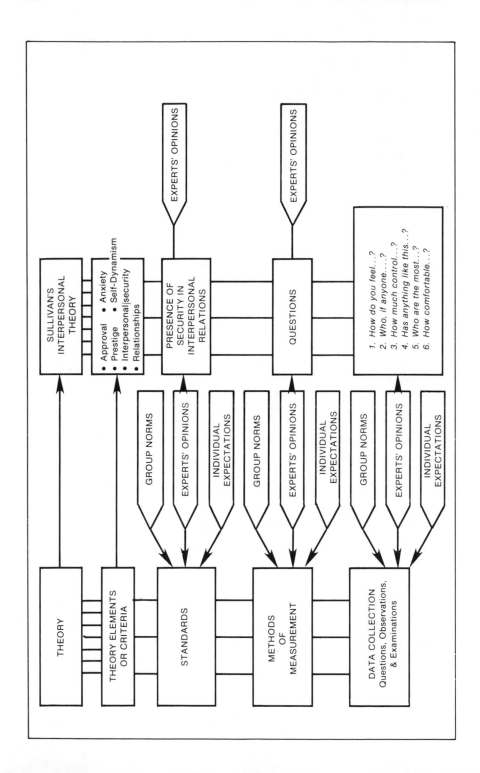

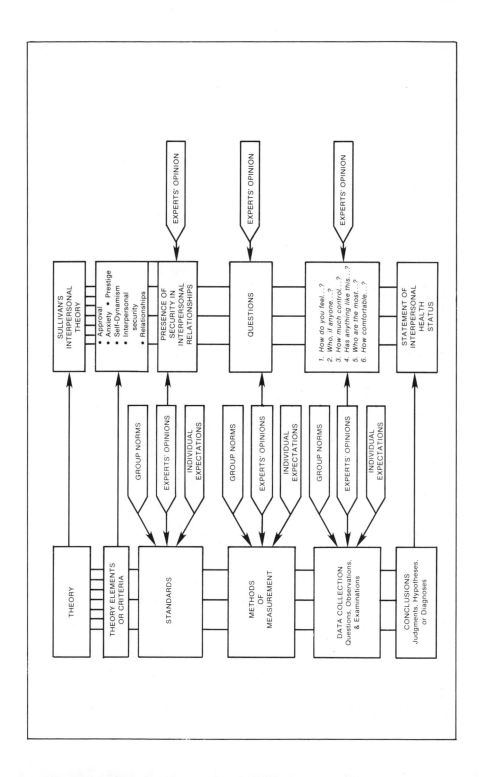

REFERENCES

1. McCain F: Nursing by assessment—not intuition. *Am J Nurs* 65:82-84, April 1965.
2. Murphy J: Toward a philosophy of nursing. In Chaska N: *The Nursing Profession: Views Through the Mist.* New York, McGraw Hill Book Co, 1978, pp 3,7.
3. McClure M: Entry into professional practice: the New York proposal. *J Nurs Adm* 6:5:12-17, June 1976.
4. Martinson I: Why research in nursing? In Chaska N: *The Nursing Profession: Views Through the Mist.* New York, McGraw Hill Book Co, 1978, pp 155-160.
5. Torres G, Yura H: *Today's Conceptual Framework: Its Relationship to the Curriculum Development Process.* New York, Department of Baccalaureate and Higher Degree Programs, National League for Nursing, 1974, pp 3-4.
6. Pinkerton A: Use of the Neuman model in a home health-care agency. In Riehl J, Roy C: *Conceptual Models for Nursing Practice.* New York, Appleton-Century-Crofts, 1974, pp 122-129.
7. Balch C: Breaking the lines of resistance. In Riehl J, Roy C: *Conceptual Models for Nursing Practice.* New York, Appleton-Century-Crofts, 1974, pp 130-134.
8. Grubbs J: An interpretation of the Johnson behavioral system model for nursing practice. In Riehl J, Roy C: *Conceptual Models for Nursing Practice.* New York, Appleton-Century-Crofts, 1974, pp 160-197.
9. Tescher B, Colavecchio R: Definition of a standard for clinical nursing practice. *J Nurs Adm* 7:32-34, 1977.
10. Kinlein M: The self-care concept. *Am J Nurs* 77:598-601, 1977.
11. Kinlein M: *Independent Nursing Practice with Clients.* Philadelphia, JB Lippincott Co, 1977.
12. Laros J: Deriving outcome criteria from a conceptual model. *Nurs Outlook* 25:333-336, 1977.
13. Jacox A: Theory construction in nursing. *Nurs Res* 23:5, 1974.
14. King I: *Toward A Theory for Nursing.* New York, Wiley and Sons, 1971, p 12.
15. Mitchell P: *Concepts Basic to Nursing.* New York, McGraw-Hill Book Co, 1973, p 137.
16. Dubin R: *Theory Building.* New York, The Free Press, 1969, pp 9,28.
17. Hardy M: Theories: components, development and evaluation. *Nurs Res* 27:100-107, 1974.
18. Douglas L, Bevis E: *Nursing Leadership in Action,* 2nd ed. St Louis, CV Mosby Co, 1974, p 2, 11.
19. Spencer M: *Contemporary Economics,* 2nd ed. New York, Worth Publishers Inc, 1974, p 5, 6.
20. Smuts J: *Holism and Evaluation.* New York, The MacMillan Co, 1926, pp 85-117.
21. Bower F: *The Process of Planning Nursing Care for Practice,* 2nd ed. St Louis, CV Mosby Co, 1977, p 11.
22. Sutterly D, Donnelly G: *Perspectives in Human Development.* Philadelphia, JB Lippincott Co, 1973, p 60.
23. Rogers M: *Theoretical Foundations for Nursing.* Philadelphia, FA Davis Co, 1970, pp 90-92, 97, 104, 113, 122.
24. Banks H: Comprehensive health planning in relation to environmental problems. *Am J Public Health* 60:10, 1973-74.
25. Branch M, Paxton P: *Providing Safe Nursing Care for Ethnic People of Color.* New York, Appleton-Century-Crofts, 1976, pp 148-150.
26. Hersey P, Blanchard K: *Management of Organization Behavior Utilizing Human Resources.* Englewood Cliffs, NJ, Prentice-Hall Inc, 1969, p 6.
27. Schulman E: *Intervention in Human Services.* St. Louis, CV Mosby Co, 1974, pp 4, 41.
28. Brennan W: The practitioner as theoretician. *Education for Social Work.* Spring 1973, p 5.

29. Maslow A: *Motivation and Personality.* 2nd ed, New York, Harper and Row, 1974.
30. Ruesch J: General theory of communication. In Arieti S (ed): *American Handbook of Psychiatry.* New York, WW Norton Inc, 1961.
31. Lewis G: *Nurse-Patient Communication.* 2nd ed, Dubuque, Iowa, Wm C Brown Co, 1973.
32. Erickson E: *Childhood and Society.* 2nd ed, New York, WW Norton, 1963.
33. Sullivan H: *Conceptions of Modern Psychiatry.* Washington, DC, William A White Psychiatric Foundation, 1947, pp 119-147.
34. Sullivan H: *The Interpersonal Theory of Psychiatry.* New York, WW Norton and Co, 1953.
35. Sullivan H: Introduction to the study of interpersonal relations. *J Psychiatry* 1:121-143, 1938.
36. Block D: Criteria, standards, norms—crucial terms in quality assurance. *J Nurs Adm* 7:7:22,pp 26-29 September 1977.
37. Stevens B: *The Nurse As Executive.* Wakefield, Mass, Contemporary Publishing Inc, 1975, pp 8, 9.
38. Bower F: Normative-or criterion-referenced evaluation? *Nurs Outlook* 22:8:499, August 1974.
39. Glasser R: Instructional technology and the measurement of learning outcomes: some questions. *Am Psychol* 17:519-521, 1963.
40. Krumme M: The case for criterion-referenced measurement. *Nurs Outlook* 23:12:764-770, December 1975.
41. Arndt C, Huckabay L: *Nursing Administration, Theory For Practice with a Systems Approach.* St Louis, CV Mosby Co, 1975, pp 144-145.
42. Brill N: *Working With People, The Helping Process.* Philadelphia, JB Lippincott Co, 1973, p 93.

BIBLIOGRAPHY

Argyris C, Schon D: *Theory in Practice: Increasing Professional Effectiveness.* San Francisco, Jossey-Bass Publishers, 1974.
Bertalanffy L: *General System Theory.* New York, George Braziller Co, 1968.
Boulding K: General systems theory—the skeleton of science. In Buckley W (ed): *Modern Systems Research for the Behavioral Scientist.* Englewood Cliffs, NJ, Prentice-Hall, 1968.
Byrne M, Thompson L: *Key Concepts for the Study and Practice of Nursing.* St Louis, CV Mosby Co, 1972.
Chater S: A conceptual framework as a basis for decisions about teaching strategies. Paper presented at *COGEN*, San Francisco, Calif, 1973.
Chater S: A conceptual framework for curriculum development. *Nursing Outlook* 23:7:425, July 1975.
Fine R: Application of leadership theory. Integrating thought and action. *Nursing Clinics of North America* 13:1:139-153, March 1978.
Fox D: *Fundamentals of Nursing Research.* New York, Appleton-Century-Crofts, 1976.
Fried E: *Ego and the Mechanisms of Defense.* New York, University Press, 1946.
Handy R: *The Measurement of Values: Behavioral Science and Philosophical Approaches.* St Louis, Warren H Green Inc, 1970.
Harms M: Development of a conceptual framework for a nursing curriculum. Paper presented at meeting of Southern Regional Education Board, Council on Collegiate Education for Nursing, Atlanta, Ga, April 9-10, 1969.
Johnson D: Development of theory: a requisite for nursing as a primary health profession. *Nursing Research* 23:5:372-377, September-October 1974.
Klein J: Theory development in nursing. In Chaska N: *The Nursing Profession: Views Through The Mist.* New York, McGraw-Hill Book Co, 1978.

Menke E: Theory development: a challenge for nursing. In Chaska N: *The Nursing Profession: Views Through The Mist.* New York, McGraw-Hill Book Co, 1978. 222.

Schlotfeldt R: Can we bring order out of the chaos of nursing education? *Am J Nurs* 76:1:105, January 1976.

Von Mering O: *A Grammar of Human Values.* Pittsburgh, University of Pittsburgh Press, 1961.

2

Assessment in Action

A nursing diagnosis is a testable conclusion or judgment derived from a systematic collection of data revealing man's health status. In effect, a nursing diagnosis represents a definable or observable point along a health-illness continuum[1,2] that describes man's ability to function in relation to theory-related standards of normalcy.[3,4] This description (diagnosis) includes a statement of the cause or precipitating factors which have affected a response. A statement of a client's health status and its cause represents a testable conclusion referred to as a nursing diagnosis. Thus, the nursing diagnosis can be classified as a hypothesis because it states predicted relationships between two variables, the health status and its cause(s).[5]

Every nursing diagnosis represents an independent function of nursing.[6,7] Each diagnosis leads to planned interventions which are predicted to bring about specific changes in the health status. A nursing diagnosis can refer to the health of an individual, a family, a group or a community.

DATA COLLECTION METHODS

In order to arrive at a nursing diagnosis, certain information must be gathered. Depending upon the source(s) of information, one or more types of data-gathering methods are employed. Sources in this context refer to the client system one is working with, the resources available, and the situation being investigated.

Questioning

Questioning is one of the most common methods of data collection and can be done verbally or in written form. Questioning is used to obtain another's perception of a situation and, therefore, represents a subjective source for obtaining information.

Questioning can take several forms, such as asking questions which are unstructured or "open-ended." Questions can also be structured to elicit specific responses such as Yes or No, or that call for a choice among suggested alternatives. Whether one decides to question verbally or in writing will depend upon the numbers and location of persons to be queried. Structured questions presume that the informant will provide information to aid in testing an already formulated theory or hypothesis. Less-structured or open-ended queries presume that one is looking for patterns in the information which would suggest a theory.[8,9] For example, the patient who has a medical diagnosis leading to a planned surgical intervention and is of a certain age group offers clear parameters indicating the use of structured questions. One source of structured questions would be standard care plans classified according to medical diagnoses. Another source might be standard care plans classified according to nursing diagnoses such as "growth and development." In the absence of patterns which suggest a theory, one asks an open-ended or "grand-tour"[4] question such as: "Can you tell me what is happening?" This type of question may be appropriate in a drop-in clinic or an emergency setting. Almost every situation in nursing, even though it may seem clearly patterned, requires "grand-tour" questions to make sure that the client's perception is heard.

Observing and Inspecting

Observing consists of looking for behavioral or situational phenomena. This form of data-gathering is needed when objective information is required to verify subjective data. It is also needed when there is no subjective data available.[10] Inspecting is one form of observation which, in the health care setting, usually refers to physical examination or clinical tests.

DEDUCTION

The process of deduction includes three sequential steps: inferring, validating, and deducing. Inferring is the formulation of several hunches, explanations, or interpretations of the data. Validation occurs when one decides what other information is needed to support or refute the initial hunches.[11,12] For example, a nurse's perception of a client's situation requires corroboration by him as part of the validation phase.[13] Finally, one comes to a conclusion (deduction) as to which hunch or inference is the defensible meaning to be drawn from the data. A conclusion describing a level of health and its causes is a nursing diagnosis.

EXPECTED VERSUS
UNEXPECTED DATA

Every client situation is laden with data or information. It is easy to become confused and frustrated in sorting out what is relevant and

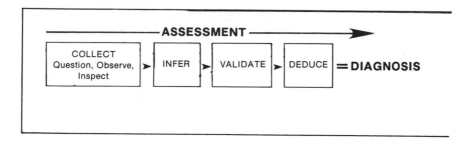

necessary to making an accurate nursing diagnosis. A helpful way out of this dilemma is to think in terms of "expected or unexpected data."

Expected Data

Expected data is what one anticipates finding in a given situation or context. Certain labels and classifications, such as a diagnosis, an age, a presenting symptom, or a need represent organizers for information. Organizers allow one to selectively choose a theory and its criteria for assessment. Suppose that a 40-year-old woman is admitted with the diagnosis of cholelithiasis. That diagnosis, her age, and sex represent organizers which allow the nurse to select diagnosis-related criteria and standards for assessment such as would be found on a pre-written standard care plan like that shown in Fig. 2.1.

The physician's diagnosis gives the nurse an organizer for the kind of data to seek and what she is likely to find. One problem to be anticipated for any patient with the diagnosis of cholelithiasis is pain. This is expected because of certain pathophysiological theories: visceral pain and referred pain. Even though a nurse can reasonably expect to find pain as an anticipated problem identified on the standard care plan, she may not always be reminded of the theories that explain the pain and its causes.

Here are examples of summarized versions of the pathophysiological theories explaining the pain associated with cholelithiasis. The term cholelithiasis implies "stones" in the gallbladder.[14]

> Most authors hypothesize a chain of events beginning with obstruction of the cystic duct or gallbladder outlet, edema due to circulatory stasis, and chemical inflammation due to stasis of bile which is irritating because of altered components.[14]

These three events result in the sensation of visceral pain, pain in the right upper quadrant radiating to the back.[15]

> Pain receptors in the visceral organs...respond only to marked changes in pressure and chemical irritants. It is also believed that in diseased visceral organs, pain results from traction, pressure, and trauma on the parietal peritoneum or on mesenteric attachments. The impulses from pain receptors

Figure 2.1

Standard Care Plan: Cholecystitis, Cholelithiasis*

DATE	USUAL PROBLEMS	EXPECTED OUTCOMES	DEADLINES	NURSING ORDERS
	1. **Pain**	1. Verbalize reasonable comfort Assist patient in position of comfort (for example semi-Fowlers)	day 2 √ q 8 hr	1. Delegate to one nurse each shift: Explore with patient his perception of pain and the illness Ascertain level of pain every 3 hours
	2. **Nausea**	2. No nausea No emesis	pre-op or day 2 √ q 8 hr	2. If needed get order for antiemetic and also explain its use to patient
	3. **Potential abdominal distention**	3. No nausea or emesis Abdomen soft and flat	day 2 √ q 8 hr	3A. If needed, get order for nasogastric tube and irrigation as needed B. Check tube for patency and proper drainage C. Palpate abdomen every 4 hours

4. Potential misunderstanding of diet at home in relation to diagnosis	4. Understanding of diet Makes correct selections from diet list	Discharge √ daily. Day Shift	4A. Have dietician see patient at least 2 days before discharge B. R.N. follow up on diet instructions
5. If patient goes to surgery, secure standard for "Cholecystectomy" to use			

*From Mayers, Mand El Camino Hospital: Standard Care Plans, *Vol. I, 1974. Courtesy of KP Medical Systems.*

in the visceral organs are conducted to the spinal cord primarily by sympathetic fibers. The cerebrum frequently misinterprets the source of pain as coming from skin surface area innervated by sensory fibers which enter the same segment of the cord as the fibers from the deep structures actually involved. This is the phenomenon of 'referred pain'.[16]

Associated with the theory of referred pain is a theory called the specificity theory.[16] This explains how pain is received in the thalmus from the visceral and skin nerve endings. In the thalmus, impulses are transferred to various parts of the cortex, resulting in the perception of pain.[17] Pain perception (threshold) tends to be the same from person to person; however, reactions to pain are extremely complex and individualized. Reactions involve the person's whole response to noxious stimuli and are determined by what the stimuli mean to him—mentally, physically, and emotionally.[17]

Again looking at expected data, it has been shown how theories of pain lead one to predict that any patient with the diagnosis of cholelithiasis will be likely to experience visceral and/or referred pain. For each of the subsequent problems appearing on the standard care plan, other theories will explain the problems or diagnoses. Using this theory-based approach to assessment, one can selectively gather data from a variety of sources: the care plan; the chart; reference books; physicians; other nurses; clients; and families. In the examples given here, the standard care plan is used as a model. There are other models which may be used or developed, such as audit criteria, flow sheets, or established assessment guides. One may start to develop assessment guides with existing models. These may, over time, be refined to include theories specific to the elements of the model. In reality, much of what nurses do is theory-based, but has not yet been clearly defined in the writing or in the thinking and dialogue of nurses. For example, the standard care plan in Fig. 2.1 does not refer to the theories. If one were to revise the pain problem, it might read: "Visceral or referred pain due to traction, pressure, and trauma."

Situations also serve as organizers for gathering expected data. For instance, patients who have sudden unplanned hospitalizations generally experience predictable problems, as do patients with recurrent admissions, or those maintained on a long-term medical regime.

Unexpected Data

Unexpected data are those for which there is no reliable framework for anticipating or predicting. These derive from less well-understood phenomena, such as the individual's values, habits, and life style. Such variables require open-ended queries to elicit the client's perceptions and those symbols which stimulate him to action.[18,4] An open-ended query is sometimes referred to as a "grand-tour" question.[4] The intent of this type of question is to learn how another person labels and defines his needs.

Grand-Tour Questions

Organizers for grand-tour questions are physiologic processes and interactions, the physical environment, and behavioral events.[4] The nurse may select any one of these organizers to begin her questioning, depending upon the situation she finds herself in with the client. She may or may not find need for all three organizers in each situation. Examples of organizers and grand-tour questions are:

Organizers	Grand-Tour Questions*
Physiological Processes and Interactions	How are you feeling?
Physical Environment	Would you show me around your home?
Behavior Events	What happened to you?

The responses to grand-tour questions will reveal the client's framework as a basis for assessment. These responses will lead to inferences relevant to that one individual. Or they can lead to the conclusion that a predetermined assessment guide is applicable in this situation. For example, if in response to the grand-tour question "How are you feeling?" the client responds by saying "I hurt all over," the nurse can pursue the client's perception of "hurting all over" by asking increasingly more specific questions, or by conducting a physiological systems review. On completing the assessment, the nurse may conclude that there is not an apparent physiological reason for the "hurt." The pain the client is feeling may be the result of an emotional turmoil he is experiencing.

In another case, in response to the same grand-tour question, the client says "I hurt right here (points to right upper quadrant of the abdomen) and in the middle of my back." This response can lead the nurse to make an assessment based on the theories of visceral and referred pain. This is an example of deciding that a predetermined assessment guide is probably applicable.

In almost every situation there is reason for using predetermined guides for assessment, as well as for posing various forms of the grand-tour question. In using both these methods of data-gathering, one must keep in mind that the assessor also has perceptions which may alter the collection and analysis of information.

---

*These are examples only. Such questions can take other forms.

INFORMATION ANALYSIS—
REVIEW AND INTERPRETATION

Analysis is the critical review and interpretation of a set of data.[19] As one reviews data, it is necessary to sort the information and discard what is irrelevant. When using predetermined standards, information is retained or discarded in accordance with the theories from which the standards were derived. In the case of the grand-tour question, one consciously sorts the information during the actual data-collection phase and retains what the patient forcefully or repeatedly emphasizes. The purpose of review-sort-discard, or retain is to extract the information crucial to further analysis.

Once review is completed, inferences can be made as to the possible meanings and relationships suggested by the information. Inferences must be validated by corroborating the nurse's tentative conclusions with the client's perceptions. When a discrepancy between the two occurs, mutual agreement must be obtained.[13] Validation thereby supports or refutes the tentative conclusions reached in the interpretation phase. If supported, one can proceed to formulate the nursing diagnosis.

DATA-GATHERING IN ACTION

Table 2.1 details man's interactive-affiliative system and is used to illustrate the standards as formulated and derived from selected theories and criteria. According to the conceptual framework in chapter 1, health is an outcome of man's reciprocal interaction with his environment. Therefore, each theory represented in the table also includes attributes of man's social/cultural environment. (Table 2.1, p. 60)

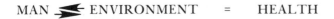

MAN   ⇌   ENVIRONMENT   =   HEALTH

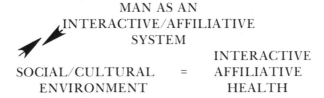

MAN AS AN
INTERACTIVE/AFFILIATIVE
SYSTEM

		INTERACTIVE
SOCIAL/CULTURAL	=	AFFILIATIVE
ENVIRONMENT		HEALTH

For purposes of illustrating the development of data-gathering guides from theories and criteria, this discussion is limited to the interactive/-affiliative theories relating to man and his social/cultural environment. If one were to develop a total assessment guide, then questions, observations, and inspections relating to all the theories of man and his environment would need to be formulated. (Table 2.1, p. 60)

It is evident from Table 2.1 that the theories, criteria, questions, and observations overlap one another. This overlap is consistent with a holistic approach to man. It can be noted that most of the interview questions are classified as grand-tour or open-ended queries. This is attributed to the fact that man is being assessed as an interactive/affiliative system and, therefore, his personal perceptions and symbols are being dealt with.

Practical Application: "Two Scenarios"

The following scenarios will illustrate two data-gathering situations between a nurse and a client, and will show how theory-related questions and observations lead to inferences. These inferences are validated with the clients and result in nursing diagnoses which describe the clients' interactive/affiliative health status.

Scenario 1

A community-health nurse is making a first prenatal visit to Janice, a 29-year-old woman. The nurse knows the client's name, age, address, referring physician, and the fact that she is two and one-half months pregnant. The nurse has entered the situation, has completed her physical assessment, and is now beginning her data-collection relating to the client's interactive/-affiliative status.

Nurse:	*Client:*
How do you feel about what's happening to you?	Oh, I feel confused, I guess, mostly upset.
Upset?	Yeah, I wish this hadn't happened. I wish I weren't pregnant right now. I'm just not ready for it.
Do you feel it's affected you — in what way?	Well, it's turned my whole life around. I really wanted to pursue my career and now it seems like I'm facing twenty years of child-raising alone.
Alone?	Yeah, I'm by myself. The father of this child, Don — he and I lived together for about two years, but after I got pregnant,

Nurse:	*Client:*
	I don't know what happened, but I'm glad he's gone; anyway, he's left.
He isn't here to help you now, then?	No.
And so you're really facing pregnancy all by yourself.	Mmmm, pregnancy and the whole future, it looks to me like.
Do you feel that you have any control over this right now?	No, that's what's so awful. I just feel a victim, like here I am pregnant. I can do something about it but I don't know if I want an abortion.
So you really don't know what you want right now?	No, it's really hard and I have to make up my mind before this goes too long, you know.
Has anything like this ever happened to you before?	Well, not quite like this before. I haven't been pregnant before.
Have you been in a situation before where you felt as if you didn't have control over what was happening to you?	Oh, gee, yes, I think so. I think a lot of my life just seems to happen by accident.
Do you remember how you felt about other situations which were similar, that you didn't have control over?	Really depressed, like I do now only it's worse now it seems.
This is the worst for you?	Yes, I know I wanted to go to college and then to have money and so I had to work. So I'm depressed about that, because I'm the victim of no money.
Are you financially secure now — you mentioned a career?	No, I don't think I'll ever be financially secure. I'm working and I manage to go to school, you know, on the side and that's been great, but now I don't know how I can manage to work and have a baby and keep going to school; you know I really wanted to be a career woman.

Nurse:	Client:
What career are you interested in?	Well, I'm interested in personnel management; I'm good at it.
And that's what you've been currently majoring in?	I'm one of the — sort of section managers of the personnel department.
Is there anyone that can be helpful to you right now, you know, who can help you right now?	Umm, my mother.
Would you still consider Don to be an important person in your life?	Yes, he's still important, but I have to let it go, you know, let that fade away.
Do you feel that you want to continue a relationship with your work people, the people that you work with?	Oh, yes, I like them, but I don't really feel comfortable about my personal life with them, you know. I've got a couple of friends, but they are not like my sister.
She's your primary person right now?	Yes, I'd say so.
In the relationships that you have with other people, do they — are they making you feel uncomfortable at this point because you're pregnant?	Well, I think that — I don't think I'm too worried about that. The people I know, my sister, and so forth, they don't seem to hold against me my being pregnant and I don't feel like that's a difficult thing.
So the people that you associate with, friends, your work relationship people, are not presenting any conflicts for you right now?	No, no.
Are there any interactions with anyone that tend to upset you right now? If Don were to come back, would that upset you?	Oh, that would really be upsetting if Don were to come around. Of course, it's upsetting not to have him around either, you know, it's bad both ways — that's upsetting.

Nurse:	*Client:*
How do you usually find out what people expect of you, for instance, in your job setting?	Well, oh, that's an interesting question. I — in my job setting I seem to function somewhat differently than I do other places, but in my job I ask and find out or double check and sometimes I guess a while and find out if I'm right or wrong, but I seem to do really well, you know. I get good evaluations, so I must get it straight.
Is it easy for you to follow through then in what you think you have to do?	At work, it is. It's easy to follow through. It's not easy — it's challenging, but I do it.
But you're able to do it?	Uhum. It's just my personal life that drives me crazy.
You don't have the same perception then about your personal life — that you do not feel as comfortable as you do — at work?	No. uhumm. My personal life keeps running into barriers and obstacles and accidents.
In the past experiences which you have had, you have been able to respond to others' expectations of you?	Ahh, that, well I —
Live up to what people think you should be doing, or job responsibilities or social obligations — feelings your family might have?	Well, I've already told you that I work. Ahh, that's OK. Ahhm — My family? I've always felt sort of the fair-haired child in my family, like everything I did was just great.
You don't feel their demands are excessive on you then?	No, I don't think so, no. That's not a problem to me. It's more maybe, well, I don't feel too secure in my social relationships outside of my family.
What about expectations for yourself? You seemed a little hard on yourself earlier when we were talking. Do you feel that you live up to your own	I don't seem to live up to any of my own. When I look back, I've always done a lot of things, but it always seems like there's a lot more that I want to accomplish,

Nurse:

expectations?

Did you live up to Don's
expectations?

It's something you mutually
experienced then?

Okay. You're really under-
going some pressures now,
talking about possible changes
in your life style and feeling a
little uncomfortable about that.

Really stressed. Were there any
ways that you've handled
pressures in the past that could
help you right now?

Is is possible that you could
use our relationship even to
talk out some of your feelings?

That's very true.

You talked to me about what
you do for your work and you
seem happy in your work life.
What do you do for leisure
time?

How do you feel about your
leisure time?

Client:

or need to, or should have. I'm
probably my own worst
taskmaster.

Well — well, I think I did pretty
well. Of course, toward the end
we both weren't living up to each
other's, and I can understand
that. You know, now looking
back on it.

Uhumm. I don't feel like there's
blame in that situation, like I
didn't do right. I didn't, but
that's not the problem.

Uhumm. More than uncomfortable — really anxious.

Well, I usually talk to people —
listen to myself talk about things
— that seems to help me decide
what to do.

I think it's possible, but of
course, I don't know you very
well.

And, uhumm, —

But I noticed your talking
today — the questions you're
asking — you know it feels kind
of good, so it's possible.

Oh, my leisure time seems to be
as busy as everything else. I seem
to — I have a lot of fun. I've
traveled quite a bit and I like
that and I like to read. I haven't
been reading much lately. What
was your question?

I feel like my leisure time is kind
of frittered away. I would like to

Nurse:	*Client:*
	use it differently. I don't exactly know how. But meanwhile it seems like I would rather just kind of float along with it.
Just let things kind of fall the way they are as far as leisure activities are concerned?	Yes, I do seem to enjoy myself, You know, I'm very active.
But you have mentioned reading and travel, so those are still current interests.	Oh, ya, uhumm.
You sort of told me many times today that you're not quite satisfied with the way your life has gone in the past, but do you feel you have some achievements?	Well actually, when I think about it — like I've gotten half-way towards my college degree by working part time. That, I think, is rather incredible.
I do too.	And I know at work I redid the whole personnel policy manual and that had needed to be done for years and no one had been able to do it; I did that. Oh, I know there are a lot of things to be proud of that I have done or can do; like I play the piano well, and I enjoy that. I think, you know, other people see me as a successful person. And, I guess, I think, I am too; I'm just very hard on myself.
Sometimes it's good to recount to other people what you have done well.	Uhumm.
Because it makes you look at your achievements — in the past and in the future too.	Right! So I suppose, you know, I can make things happen in the future. Right now, it's just that I don't know exactly what should happen.
Little too heavy? Nebulous for you right now?	Of course, if I weren't pregnant right now I know what should happen. That's my problem.
What should happen?	I should finish my degree and really move up in my career and

Nurse:

Client:

make a lot more money and do the things I like to do. It's just that, being pregnant right now, that just seems to knock it all in the head, but I just can't seem to quite face the idea of an abortion, you know? And it's really tough.

Maybe you need to know a little more about your own feelings before you can make that decision.

Yes. The more I think about my own feelings, the harder it seems. But I'm sure I have to do it.

You have mentioned being able to talk to your sister and that she is someone you can rely on and also a close relationship with your mother. Do you have easy access to these people?

Oh, my sister lives nearby and I see her almost every day if I want to. My mother is far away. Although I feel close to her, I wouldn't get into this with her, you know, I wouldn't even want her to know that I'm pregnant unless I decided to keep the baby and that's a different matter. My sister already knows I'm pregnant and knows what I'm worried about.

You mentioned that you're comfortable with your work-related people.

Uhumm.

I get the feeling that you don't have any social group ties right now — strong ties with a particular social group?

Uhumm. Not, no, except for work groups, we do things together. But outside of that, I don't. I have really been involved with Don for quite a long time and his life is very different from mine and, you know, we had a few friends together and even right now that is kind of nebulous because of us splitting up, so **I don't right now, no.**

Are your feelings and opinions about things pretty consistent with those of the people you work with?

I would say so. We have some different political views of things, but that's all right.

But you're able to meet their social expectations of you?

I think so.

Nurse:	*Client:*
How many roles do you assume right now in your life — you've already mentioned being a career girl?	Hummmm?
Student?	Oh, ya, gee. Career girl, student going to school, boss — I'm the boss of several people. Ahumm, I'm a sister. I feel like a mother already! (Nervous laughter)
Which role is the most important to you right now?	I think most important to me is maybe not any of those I mentioned, but something that has to do with me and I don't know exactly what to call that role. Maybe there isn't such a thing.
I am a person?	Something like that. I am into women's liberation a bit and, you know, the awareness of myself as a person. There's something about that, I don't know what label you put on that for a role.
What I hear you saying is that you're searching for some self-identity and that, perhaps, is the most important for you now?	That might be it. Something like that.
Are you satisfied with your performance in this world right now?	With myself?
With yourself.	Well, I am when I look at things over a time and try to be more objective about it. I'm not satisfield, though, with my dilemma.
Your current dilemma?	Uhumm.
I gather from talking to you right now that you don't have a close personal relationship with a significant person since Don has left.	No, that's another thing that I don't know about. I keep thinking that I should — want a man in my life. And that seems to be really, you know, is obviously missing right now. But my question is — Do I need a man in my life? I don't know the answer to

Nurse:	*Client:*
	that. But anyway, my sister is the person I am close to, otherwise, I don't know, I — but there seems to be something missing, you know. Maybe it's just what I'm used to — thinking I need to have a man.
You became dependent to that level that you —	Uhumm.
Having talked to you this afternoon I have just been making a few assessments of my own as to where I think you might be and I would really like to validate to see if what I've heard you say is really what you intended for me to hear you say.	Yes. Really true.
I think you've communicated very well to me that you are having some difficulties in role identity right now and experiencing some conflicts with an unwanted pregnancy.	
Umhmm, I think this is creating some uncertainty right now for you because Don has left and you're not quite sure of what your role is going to be and at no time have you mentioned talking with him about the pregnancy.	I know I haven't mentioned that. I have talked about it to him.
You have talked to him? And then that did not bring a solution for you?	No. He went into total scatter!
And that's why he's not here, right?	Uhumm.
So you're feeling a little uncertain right now about what's going to happen to you in the future?	Uhumm. Very, very uncertain.
Okay, you seem comfortable	Aha. Well, I'm not ambivalent.

Nurse:	*Client:*
in your social relationships with your peers, your work group. I felt that you were a little ambivalent in that you didn't want your mother to know about the pregnancy until you've made a decision as to whether to keep the baby or not.	I know I don't want to tell her unless it's a reality and then she'll face it with me.
But you don't feel then that that's due to a value judgment on her part — just that you want to make the decision first?	Oh, I think that she'll have some judgments, you know, she wouldn't prefer I get pregnant now, but that isn't the first time I've done something she wouldn't approve of.
But there is a lot of discrepancy there between your values and hers.	Oh, yes, I suppose so.
The other feeling I have is that you're not too satisfied with your role identity. You're a little ambivalent about that.	Especially relating to myself.
To yourself?	Uhumm.
I have the feeling that you have very high expectations and you're really not sure that you can fulfill your expectations or not; or did you talk yourself into it while we were talking?	Uhumm.
But you don't know how long that will last?	Right; it doesn't last very long.
And you are still searching for something in yourself, that would be what I would gather.	Uhumm.
Even though your sister is a good person for you to talk with right now and, if you can rely on her, I have the feeling that you're still missing a close relationship. You're not sure that you need it, but from	Yeah, that's how I'm feeling.

Nurse: *Client:*

what you've said you think
you do. Is that how you're
feeling?

Certainly you have some   I don't know — it's certainly
evidence of conflict due to   a conflict.
the unplanned pregnancy —
working with your own professional and personal goals
right now and you've not been
quite able to handle the
conflict.

Right — so your future is   Uhumm.
a little uncertain for you
right now.

I think this is probably   I feel stressed.
resulting in stress.

You feel stressed and you've   Humm. Well, I can't think of
mentioned several times you   anything else right now. I just
don't know — you're con-   need help in thinking through
sidering an abortion, but you   what to do — I have to make
don't really want an abortion   this decision.
so this is very stressful to you
right now. Is there anything
else you feel that I've missed
and that I would need to know
to help you in the next couple
of weeks when I'll be working
with you?

Relatively soon.   Uhumm.

So maybe we can proceed by   Yes, I would appreciate help
letting me come in and talk   like that.
with you and you share what
you're going through right
now. Maybe through that
process you can come to some
decision about what you
want to do.

Okay.

In this situation, the nurse did not ask every question as they appear in Table 2.1 because much of the information was offered by the client in her response to other questions. Of necessity, the questions were rephrased according to the situation and the unpredictable responses of the client. This combination of structured and open-ended questions did result in the collection of information relative to each of the elements of the interactive/affiliative theories. This information led to inferences made by the nurse, validation with the client, and nursing diagnoses. The diagnoses that emerged are theory-related. The client was given the opportunity to bring up other (unexpected) data. In this situation, none was offered. Table 2.2 shows the nurse's thought process in arriving at the nursing diagnoses. Column 1 lists the health standards derived from the theories of man's interactive/affiliative system. Column 2 reviews the information received from the client and sorts out what seems relevant. The third column shows the inferences or tentative conclusions which the nurse reached. When an inference was validated as correct, it became, in effect, the nursing diagnosis. At least two of the inferences the nurse made were not corroborated by the client. They were, therefore, rejected as diagnoses. (Table 2.2, p. 64)

Scenario 2

A staff nurse on the gynecological surgical unit is interviewing a 35-year-old married woman who is scheduled for a total hysterectomy in the morning. The nurse has introduced herself, completed the rest of the assessment, and is now ready to assess the client's interactive/affiliative health status.

Nurse:	*Client:*
Now, Mrs. Ellison, I wonder about how you're feeling — about what's happening to you right now?	I'm scared.
Scared of a —	Well, I'm scared to go to surgery and I'm not really sure what the outcome of surgery is going to be. I think I'm too young to have a hysterectomy and I really haven't been able to talk with my husband about it.
And so things seem to be happening too fast?	Seems to be going too fast! I only knew a couple of weeks ago that I was probably going to have surgery. Well, actually the doctor

Nurse:

Client:

told me a year or so ago that if
this condition didn't clear up
there was a possibility that I was
going to have surgery and I guess
I really denied the whole thing
might happen.

And now it seems to be real?

It's too real. It frightens me.

You mentioned something
about you hadn't been able to
talk about it with your
husband.

Well, every time I try to bring it
up with him, he tells me everything will work out and that's all
he ever really says, so I really
don't know how he feels about
this and it might affect our sexual
relationship; that's what I'm
really afraid of — that he might
not see me as a total woman
anymore. I don't know how I
really feel about it; I always
thought that we would have
another child and I won't be able
to after this and so it's so final.

And so it seems like, you
know, a decision has been
made that you're going to have
the surgery and you won't be
able to have a child again?

Yes.

And there's nothing you can
do about that.

No, there isn't. Of course I could
say not have the surgery and I
don't know if we could go on and
have a child or even if I could
at this point, depending on
what's wrong with me.
I'm not even sure what's wrong
with me; it's just that I'm terribly
uncomfortable and this seems to
be the only alternative I have left.
Of course, you know, the doctors
don't really explain things to you
too often either.

And so you're trusting that
what's happening, in fact,

Not very many. Maybe that's why
I'm feeling so uncomfortable

48

is a necessity?

In your feelings of discomfort with this right now and thinking about how you might deal with it, have you been in situations like this before — perhaps not like facing a hysterectomy, but other situations where you felt not in control?

So it's your health that put you in these situations.

right now. I have always been able to pretty well predict what I was going to do, and the consequences, and make a decision based on that. Only several other occasions that I can remember when I haven't been in control and, I guess, it was medically related in some way.

Yes, I have a very strong self-image that I am very healthy and until someone else convinces me otherwise, well, I get very angry both with myself and the other people.

And health has some implication — that's it, you can't change that.

Correct. And I think my husband thinks of me as strong and well. I really don't know how this is going to affect our relationship and, as I said, we haven't really talked about it; and all of a sudden tomorrow's going to be here and there's nothing we can do about it.

I hear you talk about this and I'm wondering if, since you haven't been able to talk this out with your husband and feel some reluctance to, is there anyone else who you feel is supportive to you or close to you at this time?

I've found that, since I — my family is very close to me in my own family group, my mother and sister, but they are many miles away and I have found that as I have matured and aged to the point of being 35 that our roles have changed and they have become more dependent on me. So, if there is a crisis, about the only person that I turn to is my husband.

And this time it doesn't seem quite possible at this point?

No, at this point it doesn't because I don't know if he is denying it or he truly believes that everything will be okay and my fears are unfounded, or what.

Nurse:

Client:

Or what.

Or what. I don't know.

A question again. You mentioned your mother and your sister — are there any others as important to you, are there any other people?

Not really that can help; I get a great deal of satisfaction, out of other social groups that I'm in, but when it comes to health, I feel that this is a very private concern and I'm not comfortable in discussing it with many other people.

Aha.

I would not turn to those other people for support —

Or at this point, regarding this problem.

No, no.

In terms of your life in general you mentioned other people —

Yes.

Do you work?

I do work. I work full time. I'm very active in my work. I work in one of the local libraries and I am very committed to the public. I have a son and a very active interest in his activities. These things are very important to me.

So you have work friends and colleagues.

I have work friends and then we have other social friends that come from my husband's professional relationships, plus friends that we have all gone to school together with many years ago and we're still maintaining a close relationship with them.

Of these different people that are important to you, or groups of people, which would you say is the most important — which ones?

My family.

Your family.

Definitely my family. And then I guess I have my own professional accomplishments and my peer groups that I have professional relationships with.

Nurse:	*Client:*
Okay, when you think of these people that are important to you and the groups, are there any in the past or now that you might be —	Well —
That you feel comfortable with and okay with them in terms of your fitting in or not?	Well, I feel very good about my group relationships. I guess I think sometimes their demands exceed my energy level — not my competence but my energy level, and sometimes I feel there are conflicting demands from being a wife, a mother, a professional person, and a friend. It seems that many of my friends turn to me in their times of crisis — either marital problems or health problems and often I end up — I feel supporting them and, in turn, I guess I get a little angry in that I don't think they would want to take the time to be supportive of me if I was in a comparable situation.
It feels to you that you can't rely on them; in fact you mentioned that you could not really share health problems?	That's right. I don't know if that's because they wouldn't be willing to help me or because I don't like to talk about some of my personal problems.
So you're not sure if it's them or you?	Correct.
And that doesn't —	And I wouldn't even want to do this with my sister, particularly at this time.
Are there any interactions with other people or situations that are upsetting to you or difficult to handle?	Yes, I feel very often — well, I guess I feel two things that upset me and make me a little angry. One is related to my son — he is in many groups or functions like the Boy Scouts, and school groups, and I often feel that the leaders of these groups — the other mothers have no under-

Nurse: *Client:*

standing of what my role in the community is and, therefore, ask me to do things which I have a hard time doing and it makes me angry, probably because I'm uncomfortable.

Like your energy isn't there.

Right; well, when you have a son who is active, there's a lot of responsibility. Also I feel many times — sometimes in my work setting, you know, working with young people, that their values and mine are in conflict and this sometimes creates some stress, so sometimes the job situation is stressful.

You mentioned being many things to many people — career person, mother, wife —

Friend.

Friend. Which of those roles seems the most important to you?

Well, I would say "wife" right away, but it's hard to know, and I guess it's the age-old dilemma, if you had to save your husband or child first in an accident, what would you do?

Aha.

I don't know what I would do and sometimes I'm concerned and I guess more lately than ever I have been saying to every-body, "I'm me and let me be me for awhile" instead of being wife, mother, counselor, friend or whatever. But it would come back that my family is the most important thing and I would probably sacrifice anything to maintain that role within my family.

And within your family you mentioned wife is important, and mother is important, sort of equally.

Yes.

Nurse:	*Client:*
And that really even comes before you.	Yes, which I might not like right now, but that seems to be —
What you're accepting.	For now.
In the past, well you mentioned a lot of expectations and some satisfaction with how you manage things at work; do I understand that you're satisfied with that?	Yes.
That your difficulties in working with other people may relate to your son's social groups and expectations related with that — that it's hard to meet those demands?	Well, yes, it would be very easy to have five activities a day that I was expected to participate in to meet his social demands and that sometimes makes me angry because I don't have any time left for myself —
Which is something that keeps creeping into your mind —	That's right and, I guess more than ever right now I may be feeling a little sorry for myself because I don't really understand what's happening to me here and I'm frightened, and so maybe that's making me look at other things more.
Where do you come in?	
As you're thinking about going through this possible change in your life and you don't exactly know what the change will be because of the surgery. Looking back into your past, have you dealt with similar situations — health situations — in terms of having to make some changes?	Well, yes, once, but fortunately it didn't materialize. I was told a couple of years ago that I had lumps in my breasts and it was very frightening — well, I found out it wasn't really a lump, its a — I really don't know how to explain it; it's a problem that goes away and then comes back and then goes away and then comes back, so it's never been completely resolved — so I guess there's always a little current nagging fear way back in my mind that maybe it's cancer and that they haven't really diagnosed it and now I am going to have a hysterectomy and maybe

Nurse: *Client:*

there's something they are going to find that I don't know about.

That doesn't happen to everybody, huh?

Right. And I guess maybe why my husband and I aren't talking about it is because at that time I was very frightened that I was going to lose a breast; again, we didn't talk about that too much, although I know that for me to be a desirable woman, my husband would feel that this is very important.

So it sounds like you're feeling, or you did then, that you're feeling a lot of anxiety — both of you about it.

I guess so, and I guess I'm willing to talk about it and he can't, so we're both probably feeling strained.

I would like to explore a couple of other things in terms of your leisure time in your life and so forth. I get the feeling you don't have much leisure time?

No, I find time to do things I like: I love to read, I like to dance, I like to bicycle, play tennis; I don't do those things frequently but then I don't like a lot of scheduled activities, such as "let's play tennis every Saturday morning at 8 o'clock." I like doing it, so I'm able to work that out. We do a lot of things together as a family. So we have a close family relationship.

You enjoy many of the same things together then?

Yes.

And doing it when you feel like it?

Right.

Okay, and how about your achievements in your life?
I get a feeling that you must accomplish a lot of things.

Yes, I don't feel thwarted in being able to do what I want to do and what I set out to do. I'm not through; I think I'm still a young person and I expect I'll do a lot more without any problem.

You mentioned your creeping concern for yourself and yet your really strong commit-

Uhumm.

54

Nurse:

ment to your husband and your son.

Throughout your life and as you see your life in the future, it sounds like those are close personal relationships right now and, how have you felt about your close relationships through your life?

Because it is such an important relationship?

Ahmm. Mrs. Ellison, I would like to share with you some thoughts that come to my mind in terms of where you are right now relative to your situation — your surgery — and double check with you as to whether or not my thoughts are basically correct so that if there are some things that we,

Client:

Well, I guess I went a long time in my life before I really found the person who meant a great deal to me — that being my husband, and I don't know what I would do if anything happened to that relationship right now. I feel like I'm a strong person — I feel I'm okay, but I don't know what I would do if I didn't have his support and I know we're not talking about the surgery and maybe that's what frightens me, because I don't know what our relationship will be after the surgery, although he's good. He's coming in and everything; it's not that; it's that we just can talk about everything else except when it comes to this type of situation, namely — surgery. He is so healthy that I don't know how he would really perceive me — if I couldn't do the things that I was used to doing with him or somehow his perception of me changed, I don't know what our relationship would be and that scares me.

Yes.

Yes.

Nurse:	*Client:*
here, might do, or you might do, having thought it through. I want to make sure that I'm understanding you correctly, all right?	
I'm hearing that you are frightened right now —	I am.
If you're not exactly sure of the reasons for surgery, whether it's cancer or what you've been told or understand or don't understand. I hear some fear or concern and anxiety because you need to rely on your husband and part of relying on him is talking about this.	Right.
And so that's a concern; and another thing I understand is that you do have a close relationship with your husband — meaningful and important. You rely on that a lot.	That's true. He's my outlet; it's through him that I get rid of my other feelings or can handle them or whatever.
And so you have a real strength there — an importance in that relationship. I understand also that in terms of your life in general, you feel good about your friends and the people and the groups that you relate to and work with and feel good about meeting their expectations.	Uhumm.
And values and that, generally, you are able to do what you want to do?	Generally, right.
That you usually feel in control of your life and there's been only a couple of times	Yes, I guess that's what is so frightening; I don't like that feeling.

Nurse:	Client:
in your life that you haven't — this being one of them?	
And those are some of the **main things that I under-**stand from the things you've shared about your situation. I wonder if there's anything else that perhaps comes into your mind that you haven't had a chance to mention?	I don't think so — I guess I'm just so — aah, I don't like surgery anyhow. The very fact that I'm going to have surgery frightens me and then the fact that is unknown right now and I really don't know how my husband feels is what's really bothering me.
That seems to be your main concern.	Right.
Since it does seem to be a real concern to you, one of the things that I or my colleagues might be able to offer you is some help in figuring out what to do about it, even though you do have what seems to be a very short time frame before tomorrow morning.	I guess they expect us to come in and have surgery and everything will be okay and until you've had surgery yourself, it's a frightening experience — it really is.
We might take the next step in deciding what to do about it. I'll be back before visiting hours to see if there's any way you can approach your husband on the subject.	Okay.

Table 2.3 (p. 67) shows the thought process reflected in this scenario when assessing Mrs. Ellison's interactive/affiliative health status.

The diagnoses in the right-hand column of Table 2.3 are again theory-related. This scenario reflects the use of the same basic questions, but focuses on the concerns a client might experience in a physician's acute care setting. The questions may vary according to the situation in which the data-gathering is done. The client's response may also vary according to his perception of the situation. Clients' responses may also be altered by nurses' own values and preconceived ideas stemming from their own life experiences. To minimize the risk of misinterpreting the patient's behavior and creating problems which actually don't exist, it is essential to validate inferences with the client before coming to conclusions or diagnoses.

For example, in the first scenario, the nurse, because of her own feelings about herself and her relationship with her mother, experienced strong feelings that Janice was having difficulty telling her mother of the pregnancy due to fear of rejection, "discrepancy in values." When the nurse went back to validate this perception, Janice insisted that she felt confident her mother would not be rejecting but would be very supportive of her. This inferencing and validation process is reflected in items 6 and 10 on the table on page   . The table shows that the nurse changed her tentative diagnosis after checking with the client. The table also shows that validation supported some of the nurse's initial inferences.

In the second scenario, the nurse imposed her own opinions in making the inference that the patient was self-sacrificing to her own detriment. Upon validating this with Mrs. Ellison, she reconfirmed her previous statements that this was not a problem which she chose to pursue. Further validation revealed that the nurse's inference that the husband was supportive was not perceived to be correct by the client. This led the nurse to reject this inference and to make a nursing diagnosis consistent with the client's view.

After the nurse left the room, the client was still concerned about her real fears of having to have a general anesthesia in the morning and her fear over changes in self-image due to a degenerative arthritis. These fears were left unexplored by the nurse, possibly because of her bias as to what the immediate problem was and the fact that she experienced some anxiety during the interview. This made the nurse feel uncomfortable, resulting in her terminating the interview without offering Mrs. Ellison a chance to explore other concerns.

In both of the patient situations described, if the nurse had not validated her inferences she would have imposed her values on the client by either missing problems or identifying problems which did not exist. Despite validation, the nurse's mind-set in the second scenario caused her to preclude identifying additional concerns of the client.

Interactive/Affiliative
Assessments in a
Variety of Settings

The degree to which the interactive/affiliative system, or any system, is explored and assessed depends upon the variables in a given situation; the physician's diagnosis, the presenting problem, the person or persons involved, the time element, and the setting.

The Rapid-Care Setting—In the emergency department, the focus of care is on the immediate situation and usually relates to critical physical needs. Thus, it may not generally be appropriate to assess a person's interactive/affiliative health status if physical survival needs are the priority. On the other hand, the ability of the client and his family or significant others to adapt to the immediacy of the situation will need to be assessed. The nurse may need to assume a supportive role in helping both the client and his family to interact effectively with one another and with the personnel in the rapid-care setting. The same principles are appropriate in an intensive- or critical-care unit.

Extended-Care Setting—In long-term care settings, strong emphasis should be placed on client's interactive/affiliative systems, both with their social needs within the institution as well as with those outside the institution. Their interactive/affiliative needs must be assessed and supported through the nursing process. Both clients and nurses run the risk of becoming victims to mind-sets that may violate the individual's interactive/affiliative needs. Assessment of this system is necessary for maintaining social viability of the client's health status. Similar principles apply to clients in a mental-health setting. Deficiencies in meeting interactive/affiliative needs may be the precipitating cause of many mental-health problems and crises.

THEORY—BASED ASSESSMENT

This entire chapter has illustrated the process of deriving assessment criteria from theories, developing assessment guides from criteria, assessing a client, and formulating nursing diagnoses consistent with theory. This has been done within the context of the conceptual framework presented in the first chapter. A set of theories related to man as an interactive/affiliative system was chosen for use. This system represents one of the seven systems which interpret man in the conceptual framework. Each of the other systems suggests theories and lends itself to the same process. Theory-related criteria and standards from all six systems provide the basis for a complete set of assessment criteria. Appendix A shows data-collection guides for the remaining systems of man.

It becomes evident as one explores the six systems of man that many theories overlap; thus, criteria and standards may overlap from system to system. In the data-gathering process, a complete set of data-collection guides can be utilized which together are representative of all six systems. It is also evident that client situations do not present themselves in pure theoretical form, again creating the necessity for flexibility across systems. In some situations, some criteria are more relevant than others or may require a different focus of attention. However, the overlapping of systems, theories, questions, observations, and nursing diagnoses is consistent with the holistic view of man. Theory-based decision-making is consistent with a scientific and humanistic nursing process.

Although this chapter has focused primarily on "intake" or preliminary assessment processes, the same priniciples apply in the ongoing process of client-centered care on a daily basis. Theory-based intake standards provide baseline data for subsequent progress evaluation and for eliciting new information as the client situation changes. This ongoing analysis of the client situation using theory-based criteria provides the basis for documentation of the client's status.

Table 2.1

Man as an Interactive/Affiliative System

THEORIES	CRITERIA	HEALTH STANDARDS	METHODS OF MEASUREMENT	DATA COLLECTION: QUESTIONS, OBSERVATIONS, EXAMINATIONS

Interpersonal Theories
Sullivan[20,21,22] Tension reduction and security combine to become the major behavior goals of any individual. These goals require feelings of approval and prestige. A person's self-concept or self-dynamism organizes behavior and is a result of past and present experiences with significant others. Behavior, emotions and needs originate from the interaction of one individual with another. Anxiety is the chief disruptive force in interpersonal relationships. Interpersonal security is a major human need. Past relationships influence perceptions of present relationships.
 	
Insecurity in interpersonal relationships produces anxiety.
	Feelings of approval
	
	Feelings of prestige
	
	Anxiety, tension
	
	Self-dynamism, self-concept
	
	Interpersonal security
	
	Perceptions of past and present relationships/ interactions
		Presence of feelings of security in most important interpersonal relationships	Structured and nonstructured questions	*Questions*
				How do you feel about what is happening to you?
				   Put down
				   Not recognized or valued
				
				Do you feel you have control over what is happening to you?
				
				Has something like this ever happened before?
				   What do you remember about it?
				
				Who, if anyone, can help you (be supportive to you) at this time?
				
				Who are the important people in your life?
				   Family
				   Significant others
				   Work group
				   Social group

A person will interact to reduce anxiety. Present interactions are influenced by perceptions of past interactions.				Do relationships with these people make you feel comfortable/uncomfortable?
Communication Theories				
Reusch[23] Communication results when one mind is able to affect another. Transmitting, receiving, and validating are necessary for communication.	Behavior change: self — others Information processing	Ability to change behavior of self or others in an attempt to reduce uncertainty.	Structured and nonstructured questions. Observations	*Questions* How do you usually find out what others expect of you? How easy or difficult is it for you to follow through? In your past, how have you been able to respond to your own or others' expectations? Do you usually feel in control of the situation, or a victim of the circumstances?
Bevis[24] Human productivity and survival are dependent upon communication-interpersonal, intrapersonal, and community.	Productivity	Ability to communicate in interpersonal and group relationships.	Structured and nonstructured questions. Observations	How have you generally responded to pressures for change in your life style? What type of work do you do? How do you feel about your achievements in life? What important things do you feel you have accomplished?

THEORIES	CRITERIA	HEALTH STANDARDS	METHODS OF MEASUREMENT	DATA COLLECTION: QUESTIONS, OBSERVATIONS, EXAMINATIONS
Group Role Theory Robbins[25] How a person behaves is determined by the role defined in a given context. When a group exists, role perceptions and expectations exist. Role conflict occurs when one or more group(s) expectations cannot be met. Lost roles lead to identity problems. Lost roles if replaced minimize identity crisis.[26]	Social Kin networks[27]	Membership in one or more social groups. Membership in a kin network. Perceived sense of comfort with values and norms of reference groups. Ability to rank loyalties among reference groups. Satisfaction with role identity.	Structured and nonstructured questions. Observations	*Observations* Transmitting ideas clearly. Receiving or understanding. Validating or checking out. *Questions* Is there someone/s on whom you rely? How easy is it to keep in touch with those who are important to you? What groups are you affiliated with? Which do you feel most comfortable with? How consistent are your opinions and feelings with those in the group? Which groups are the most important to you? How able are you to meet their expectations?

				How many roles do you assume right now in your life? Which role is most important? Are you satisfied with this role? *Observations* Body language Posture Muscle tension Facial expressions Random/compulsive movements Tone of voice
Intimacy Theory Angyal[28] The maintenance of closeness with another is the center of existence up to the very end of life.	Intimacy	Closeness with another throughout life.	Nonstructured questions	*Questions* What about close personal relationships in your life?
Culture Theory Robbins[25] Mead[29] Sumner[30] Man's needs, wishes, desires, value systems and behavior norms are determined by reference groups.	Values, behaviors and goals	State of being consistent with the values, norms and goals of the most important reference groups.	Structured and nonstructured questions Observations	Refer to previous questions relative to Group/Role.

Table 2.2

Nursing Diagnoses, Scenario One

HEALTH STANDARDS	DATA REVIEW	INFERENCES	VALIDATION: NURSING DIAGNOSES
HEALTH IS: 1. Presence of feelings of security in most important interpersonal relationships	Secure in work groups and with sister. Social group not important now. Construes self to be inadequate even though others give positive feedback.	Not okay. Constant insecurity due to conflict between self-expectations and achievements and decision to terminate pregnancy.	Correct
2. Ability to change behavior of self or others in an attempt to reduce uncertainty	History of validating groups' perceptions of self, expectations of self and responsibilities. Can function in directing and supervising others. Able to work and go to school concurrently.	OK	Correct
3. Ability to communicate in interpersonal and group relationships	See above. Also, able to communicate in interview session.	OK	Correct
4. Membership in one or more social groups	Socializes with members of work group only.	OK	Correct
5. Membership in a kin network	Feels close to mother and sister.	OK	Correct
6. Perceived sense of comfort with values and norms of reference groups	States unwillingness to tell mother about pregnancy unless she has to.	Not ok. Potential conflict with mother due to violating mother's values, fear of rejection	Not correct — client is in a healthy state.

7. Ability to rank loyalties among reference groups.	States comfortableness with friends — minor political differences of no consequence. She and mother's values not always consistent but mother will stand by her	OK	Correct
	Limited reference — thus no expressed difficulty — or conflict between work and family	OK	Correct
8. Satisfaction with role identity.	In conflict with unwanted pregnancy. Struggles with self-identity as a woman alone — questioning wanting or needing dependence on man.	Not okay. Sudden role ambivalency due to unwanted pregnancy.	
	Relates satisfaction with role of boss, sister, student — already feels like a mother. States career goals.		
	Observation: Hands clasped tightly...long heavy sigh... occasional posture change from relaxed position to upright. Frequent movement of hands/feet.		

Table 2.2 *(cont.)*
Nursing Diagnoses, Scenario One

HEALTH STANDARDS	DATA REVIEW	INFERENCES	VALIDATION: NURSING DIAGNOSES
9. Closeness with another throughout life.	History of intimate relationship with one person. Now experiencing a loss of that relationship. Questioning future close relationship of similar nature.	Not okay. Uncertainty due to change in future role and establishing a relationship with another man.	Correct
10. State of being consistent with the values, norms, and goals of most important reference groups.	See item 6.	See item 6.	Not correct. See item 6. Client is in a healthy state.

Table 2.3
Nursing Diagnoses, Scenario Two

HEALTH STANDARDS	DATA REVIEW	INFERENCES	VALIDATION: NURSING DIAGNOSES
HEALTH IS: 1. Presence of feelings of security in most important interpersonal relationships	Several interpersonal relationships — none causing severe stress or presenting problems which can't be dealt with.	OK	Correct
2. Ability to change behavior of self or others in an attempt to reduce uncertainty	General ability to influence others and change in accordance with others' expectations: child's expectation, husband's professional group's expectations.	OK	Correct
3. Ability to communicate in interpersonal and group relationships	See item 1. In interview articulate, verbal, expressing self well	OK	Correct
4. Membership in one or more social groups	Mention of work friends, old school friends, social and professional relationships	OK	Correct
5. Membership in kin network	Strong, close family relationship with husband, son, parents and sister	OK	Correct

Table 2.3 *(cont.)*
Nursing Diagnoses, Scenario Two

HEALTH STANDARDS	DATA REVIEW	INFERENCES	VALIDATION: NURSING DIAGNOSES
6. Perceived sense of comfort with values and norms of reference groups	Great loyalty to family — states "they come first." Work group important. Referred to other social group. Satisfied with current roles in groups.	OK	Correct
7. Ability to rank loyalties among reference groups	Definitely ranks family first. Some frustration regarding loyalties to other reference groups.	OK	Correct
8. Satisfaction with role identity	Some ambivalence regarding satisfaction or sacrifice of personal needs to meet needs of family. Willingness to defer this concern at this time but hint of concern regarding own perception of self or change due to surgery.	Not okay. Suppressing own emotional needs due to family demands.	Not correct

9. Closeness with another throughout life	Close, strong basic relationship with husband. Strong needs to rely on husband. Inability to talk about implications of this surgery with husband. Statement that if anything happened to relationship, "don't know what I would do." *Observation:* Speech very rapid without pauses. Otherwise throughout interview voice tone calm and well controlled. Posture unchanged. Tendency to look straight ahead rather than at interviewer.	OK	Not correct — Acute fear due to unknowns regarding husband's feelings and relations and due to uncertainty of outcome of surgery.
10. A state of being consistent with the values, norms, and goals of most important reference groups	See item 6.	See item 6.	

REFERENCES

1. Dunn H: What high level wellness means. *Can J Public Health* 50:444-457, 1959.
2. Byrne M, Thompson L: *Key Concepts for the Study and Practice of Nursing.* St Louis, CV Mosby Co, 1972, p 33.
3. Friedson E: *A Profession of Medicine.* New York, Dodd Mead and Co, 1970.
4. Spradley J, McCUrdy D: *The Cultural Experience: Ethnography in Complex Society.* Chicago, Science Research Association, Inc, 1972, pp 22-38, 61, 62, 68.
5. Notter L: *Essentials of Nursing Research.* New York, Springer Publishing Co, Inc, 1974, p 142.
6. Bernzweig E: *The Nurse's Liability for Malpractice,* 2nd ed. New York, McGraw Hill Book Co, 1975, pp 114-115.
7. Lesnick M, Anderson B: *Nursing Practice and the Law.* Philadelphia, JB Lippincott Co, 1962, p 270.
8. Brill N: Working with People, *The Helping Process.* Philadelphia, JB Lippincott Co, 1973, p 71.
9. Glasser B, Strauss A: *The Discovery of Grounded Theory: Strategies for Qualitative Research.* Chicago, Aldine Publishing Co, 1967.
10. Larkin P, Bacher B; *Problem-Oriented Nursing Assessment.* New York, McGraw Hill Book Co, 1977, p 4.
11. Schulman E: *Intervention in Human Services.* St Louis, CV Mosby Co, 1974, pp 36-39.
12. Bailey J, Claus K: *Decision Making in Nursing, Tools for Change.* St Louis, CV Mosby Co, 1975, pp 10-14.
13. Marriner A: *The Nursing Process, A Scientific Approach to Nursing Care.* St Louis, CV Mosby Co, 1975, pp 9-11.
14. Luckmann J, Sorenson K: *Medical-Surgical Nursing, A Psychophysiologic Approach.* Philadelphia, WB Saunders Co, 1974, p 1136.
15. Beyers M, Dudas S: *The Clinical Practice of Medical-Surgical Nursing.* Boston, Little-Brown and Co, 1977, p 605.
16. Shafer K, et al: *Medical-Surgical Nursing,* 6th ed. St Louis, CV Mosby Co, 1975, p 164.
17. Crawley D: *Pain and Its Alleviation.* Berkeley, Calif, University of California, 1962, pp 16, 22.
18. Day R: *Perception.* Dubuque, Iowa, William C Brown Co, 1966, pp 6-9, 34, 42, 43.
19. Mayers M, Norby R, Watson A: *Quality Assurance for Patient Care: Nursing Perspectives.* New York, Appleton-Century-Crofts, 1977, p 57.
20. Sullivan H: Conceptions of Modern Psychiatry. Washington, DC, William A White Psychiatrics Foundation, 1947, pp 119-147.
21. Sullivan H: The Interpersonal Theory of Psychiatry. New York, WW Norton and Co, Inc, 1953.
22. Sullivan H: Introduction to the study of interpersonal relations. *J Psychiatr* 1:121-134, 1938.
23. Reusch J: General Theory of Communication. In *American Handbook of Psychiatry,* New York, WW Norton and Co, Inc, 1961.
24. Bevis E: *Curriculum Building in Nursing, a Process.* St Louis, CV Mosby Co, 1973, p 75.
25. Robbins S: *The Administrative Process, Integrating Theory and Practice.* Englewood Cliffs, NJ, Prentice-Hall, Inc, 1976, pp 283-284, 23-29, 34.
26. Miller S: The social dilemma of the aging leisure participant. In Doser A, Peterson W, (eds): *Older People and Their Social World.* Philadelphia, FA Davis Co., 1965.
27. Sussman M (ed): *Source Book In Marriage and the Family.* New York, Houghton Mifflin Co, 1963.
28. Angyal A: *Neurosis and Treatment: A Holistic Theory.* New York, John Wiley and Sons, Inc, 1965.

29. Mead M (ed): *Cultural Patterns and Technical Change*. New York, UNESCO, A Mentor Book, 1955, pp 12-13.

30. Sumner W: *Folkways*. New York, Ginn, 1906.

BIBLIOGRAPHY

Anthony W, Carkhuff R: *The Art of Health Care*. Amherst, Mass. Human Resource Development Press. 1976.

Atchley R: Retirement and leisure participations: continuity or crisis? *Gerontologist* 11:13-17, 1971.

Bailey J, Claus K: *Decision Making in Nursing, Tools for Change*. St Louis, CV Mosby Co, 1975.

Barnlund D: Toward a meaning-centered philosophy of education. *ETC: A Review of General Semantics*, December 1963.

Beeson P, McDermott W: *Textbook of Medicine*, 14th ed. Philadelphia, WB Saunders Co, 1975.

Beland I, Passas J: *Clinical Nursing, Pathophysiological and Psycho-social Approaches*, 3rd ed. New York, McMillan Publishing Co, Inc, 1975.

Berlo D: *The Process of Communication*. New York, Holt, Rinehart and Winston, Inc, 1960.

Berni R, Readey H: *Problem-Oriented Medical Record Implementation: Allied Health Peer Review*. St Louis, CV Mosby Co, 1974.

Bower F: *The Process of Planning Nursing Care, A Model For Practice*, 2nd ed. St Louis, CV Mosby Co, 1977.

Brill N: Teamwork: *Working Together in the Human Services*. Philadelphia, JB Lippincott Co, 1976.

Byrne M, Thompson L: *Key Concepts for the Study and Practice of Nursing*. St Louis, CV Mosby Co, 1972.

Clark M: The anthropology of aging: a new area for studies of culture and personality, *Gerontologist* 7, March 1967.

Creighton H: *Law Every Nurse Should Know*, 3rd ed. Philadelphia, WB Saunders Co, 1975.

Douglas L, Bevis E: *Nursing Leadership in Action*, 2nd ed. St Louis, CV Mosby Co, 1974.

Fox D: *Fundamentals of Research in Nursing*, 3rd ed. New York, Appleton-Century-Crofts, 1976.

Gebbie K, Lavin M (eds): Classification of nursing diagnosis. In *Proceedings of the First National Conference*, St Louis, CV Mosby Co, 1975.

Gragg S, Reese O: *Scientific Principles in Nursing*, 7th ed. St Louis, CV Mosby Co, 1974.

Hagen E: Conceptual issues in the appraisal of the quality of care. In *Assessment of Nursing Services*, Bethesda, Md, US Department of Health, Education, and Welfare, June 1974, pp 49-76.

Hymovich D, Barnard M: *Family Health Care*. New York, McGraw-Hill Co, 1977.

Lambertson E: *Education for Nursing Leadership*. Philadelphia, JB Lippincott Co, 1958.

Laxton D, Hyland P: *Planning and Implementing Nursing Intervention*. St Louis, CV Mosby Co, 1975.

Leininger M: The culture concept and its relevance to nursing. In Auld M, Birum L (eds): *The Challenge of Nursing, A Book of Readings*, St Louis, CV Mosby Co, 1973, pp 39-46.

Lewis G: *Nurse-Patient Communication*. Dubuque, Iowa, William C Brown Co, 1973.

Little D, Carnevali D: *Nursing Care Planning*, 2nd ed. Philadelphia, JB Lippincott Co, 1976.

Mager R, Pipe P: *Analyzing Performance Problems*. Belmont, Calif, Lear Siegler Inc, Fearon Publishers, 1970.

Mayers M: *A Systematic Approach to the Nursing Care Plan*. New York, Appleton-Century-Crofts, 1972.

Mitchell P: *Concepts Basic to Nursing*, 2nd ed. New York, McGraw-Hill Book Co, 1977.

Mundinger M, Jauron G: Developing a nursing diagnosis. *Nurs Outlook* 23:94-98, February 1975.

Neugarten B, Moore J, Lowe J: Age norms, age constructs and adult socialization. *Am J Sociol* 70:6, May 1965.

Notter L: *Essentials of Nursing Research*. New York, Springer Publishing Company, Inc, 1974.

Rose A: A systematic summary of symbolic interaction theory. In Riehl J, Roy C: *Conceptual Models for Nursing Practice*, New York, Appleton-Century-Crofts, 1974, pp 34-46.

Roy C: A diagnostic classification system for nursing. *Nurs Outlook* 23:90-94, February 1975.

Ryan B: Nursing care plans: a system approach to developing criteria for planning and evaluating. *J Nurs Adm* 3:50, May-June 1973.

Sarbin T: The scientific status of the mental-illness metaphor. In Plag S, Edgerton R (eds): *Changing Perspectives in Mental Illness*, New York, Holt, Rinehart and Winston, 1969, pp 23-24.

Stevens B: *The Nurse as Executive*. Wakefield, Mass, Contemporary Publishing Co, 1975.

Stone S, et al (eds): *Management for Nurses, A Multidisciplinary Approach*. St Louis, CV Mosby Co, 1976.

Sumner W, Keller A, Davil M: *The Science of Society*. New Haven, Conn, Yale University Press, 1917.

Systematic Nursing Assessment: *A Step Toward Automation*. Washington, DC, State University of New York at Buffalo, Faculty of Health Sciences, National Institutes of Health, December 1971.

Treece E, Treece J: *Elements of Research in Nursing*, 2nd ed. St Louis, CV Mosby Co, 1977.

Walter J, Pardu G, Malbo D (eds): *Dynamics of Problem-Oriented Approaches: Patient Care and Documentation*. Philadelphia, JB Lippincott Co, 1976.

Watson A, Mayers M: *Care Planning: Chronic Problem, Stat Solution*. Stockton, Calif, KP Company Medical Systems, 1976.

Yura H, Walsh M: *The Nursing Process: Assessing, Planning, Implementing, Evaluating*, 2nd ed. New York, Appleton-Century-Crofts, 1973.

3

Documentation in Action

Documentation is the act of assembling, coding, and disseminating information in written form. It provides factual or substantial support for statements made or for hypotheses proposed.[1] Written documentation preserves for historical reference the facts and evidence of the nursing process and the clients' responses. This statement raises a question: *Which facts and what substantial evidence are important to preserve?*

Within the context of this text, it is suggested that the conceptual framework provides the guide for determining what facts and evidence need to be assembled, coded, and disseminated.

ASSEMBLING, CODING, AND DISSEMINATING INFORMATION

Assembling

Assembling information means to collect it into one or more appropriate places. It also implies classifying information and relating the classifications to one another in a logical fashion. Assembling of information means, then, that one must decide where information is to be located: What information should be on a rand, in the patient record, on the care plan, in a computer memory bank, on microfilm, in a file, or simultaneously in many departments or places? It also raises questions such as: How should information be classified? Should it be classified by medical diagnosis, by chronological flow of events, by nursing unit, or by types of events? Other questions relate to how all this information gets together. What needs to be duplicated? What category of information relates to another? What overlaps with another? What needs to be condensed and summarized for easy analysis? What disciplines need to contribute jointly?

Coding

Coding is the act of devising a system of principles, rules, and signals for communication of information. To devise a coding system, many things must be considered. What do regulatory bodies require for licensing, accreditation, certification, reimbursement, utilization review, and quality monitoring? What do laws regarding freedom of information and confidentiality require? What do the nurse's insurance carrier and legal advisor insist upon? What do the nurse's philosophy and her conceptual framework mandate?

Disseminating

Disseminating is the process of reporting, circulating, and retrieving the right information to and from the right people and places. This process holds information for the future. To activate this process, one needs to consider the following questions: Who needs what information and when? How best is the information dispersed—on a form, in a letter, in a progress note, on a tape, on a transcriber, in a computer? What information needs to be stored and for how long? When should the information be stored? How can information be retrieved? Who does the information belong to—the staff, the nurse, the director of nursing, the agency, the client? Who is responsible to act on the information? What information is confidential? Are there degrees of confidentiality? What information is privileged? What informtion must be made public? How can information be made legible and understandable? Almost none of these questions can be answered without some reference to a conceptual framework.

THE CONCEPTUAL FRAMEWORK
AS AN AID
TO DOCUMENTATION

A conceptual framework and its components aid substantially in establishing the documentation process. It is particularly helpful for the coding and classifying of information. A conceptual framework insures that the pieces of documentation fit together, thereby reducing omissions and preventing duplication. A conceptual framework also establishes what facts and substantial evidence are needed to support statements and hypotheses about man and his environment. The theories provide the supporting assumptions and logic that underline documented facts and statements about health. The concepts of nursing—human, conceptual, and technical—guide documentation about man (the client) and the environment and how they interact to achieve or maintain health.

Nursing, as an open system, cannot be divided into three discrete functions; they overlap one another and are used simultaneously to assess man and the environment. The concept of human function refers to nursing as an interactive process; therefore this aspect of the process must be included as a component in the documentation system. The conceptual function of nursing defines the decision process; thus the logic for decisions must appear either directly or indirectly in the document. Similarly, the technical function of nursing with its technological, administrative, educational, and research components provides the guidelines, rules, and exceptions for the implementation and documentation of nursing practice at all levels.

Questions relative to the assembling of information can best be answered by reviewing the concept of nursing as a technical function. Specifically, administration, a process of planning, directing, organizing, controlling, and evaluating, leads to decisions as to where, how, when, and by whom information should be recorded. For instance, all elements of administration use decision-making as a guiding theory. The directing element of administration is responsible for a philosophy and for selection of goals. The planning element, in relationship to the philosophy and purposes, encompasses issues, "problems" to be resolved, isolation of fact from fiction, determination of goals and possible alternatives, and then selection of the most defensible alternatives. Whether one is a member of a faculty group in a school of nursing, of a management group in a health-care service, of colleagues in a research situation, or of staff nurses providing direct care, it is essential that he use the administrative process to determine the documentation system as a whole with component parts. Education and research also influence how information is assembled, coded, and disseminated.

The conceptual function of nursing assists in making decisions about classification schemes. Concepts and related theories from one's conceptual framework provide the intellectual basis and the organizers for classifying information so that nursing practice can be analyzed and evaluated.

Coding

A documentation system includes principles, rules, and symbols for communicating in writing. Principles are derived from one's beliefs and interpretations of nursing as a construct in relation to man and his reciprocal relationship with the environment. Rules generally are arbitrary and are imposed or agreed upon through such external and internal regulatory mechanisms and groups as state licensing boards and organization policies. Communication signals are symbols which convey a universal meaning. A rather standard example is a list of accepted abbreviations. Most documentation systems require a stated coding system to minimize error, increase efficiency, and reduce cost.

Disseminating

Dissemination is the process of determining the best or most appropriate channels for reporting, circulating, and retrieving information. Channels are both formal and informal and are established by the group, the organization, or the care giver, and the client. For documentation purposes, formal communication, is here limited to groups and organizations, channels traditionally following an authority network. Between a professional and a client or a group of clients, channels of communication are negotiated. Communication channels must include a feedback mechanism to validate that the message received was the same as that sent. More specifically, in formal groups and organizations, communication can flow downward, upward, laterally (horizontally) and externally. "Superior-subordinate interaction represents a downward communication flow..."[2] such as instructions and policy. "When subordinates initiate communications to their superiors, the flow is upward, and the messages may include participation in decision-making, expressions of dissatisfaction, or opinions and, most important, they may provide evaluative input on individual and unit performance."[2] Lateral communications are usually designed to coordinate intergroup activities. These may include memos, minutes, or reports between faculty members or departments, between hospital staff or patient-care units, or between client and provider. Finally, documentation flows externally from the person, the group, or the organization to someone outside of the system. This may take the form of a referral to another agency, a report to a government agency, a proposal to a community group, or a letter to a client. Decisions about communication channels can be derived from all three functions of nursing: human, conceptual, and technical.

METHODS OF DOCUMENTATION

Client-centered documentation within nursing service generally can be seen to take one or a combination of three forms: source-oriented; problem-oriented; and outcome-oriented. For the purpose here the focus is on client-centered documentation. Written communication systems for educational settings or for service settings are being described.

Source-Oriented

Source-oriented records[3] refer to a method of categorizing client information according to the discipline or department which provides the data. This is a traditional and familiar form of record-keeping and is especially noticeable in a chart where one finds separate sections for physicians' orders, nurses' notes, laboratory results, x-ray results, and separate sections for other classifications. An advantage of this method is that it is easy to find one's own section and to chart accordingly. The disadvantage lies in the retrieval of information. Obviously it is necessary to look at several or all sections of the chart to gain relevant information about even one problem or issue. A further disadvantage, either by design or default, is that each discipline uses its own coding system, systems which other disciplines may not understand.

Problem-Oriented

Problem-oriented records differ from source-oriented records in that they are organized according to a list of the client's problems. The list becomes the index for subsequent classification, input, and retrieval of information. It provides for the integration of information from all disciplines providing care to the client. "The emphasis is not on who gives the care but on the problems for which the care is given."[3] Many modifications for this documentation method have been developed; however, the original system was introduced by Lawrence Weed.[4] The original system contains four major components: data base, problem list, initial plan, and progress notes.

Data Base

The data base is generated from many sources and is a systematic compilation of information that assists the various professionals to diagnose the client's problems. The systematic data-gathering guide includes:

1. *Historical*
   - ID — Identification: demographic and administrative data (name, age, address, insurance information, etc.)
   - PH — Past History: medical-surgical, allergic problems, hospitalizations, previous exams and tests, dental records, eye records, etc.
   - RX — Past and current treatment, immunizations, coffee, cigarette and drug usage, etc.
   - FH — Family History: genetic and medical.
   - SH — Social History (patient profile): habits, hobbies, recreations, activities, family situation, economic status, education, jobs, profile of typical day, religion, personal strengths and preferences, etc.
   - ROS — Review of Systems: structured review of body systems relative to symptoms or possible problems.
2. *Physiological*
   Body measurements (height, weight, etc.), vital signs (heart rate,

blood pressure, etc.), general physical examination (not including details on problems).

3. *Laboratory*

Routine tests such as blood chemistry ("battery"), "hemogram," urinalysis, chest x-ray, EKG, PAP smear.[5]

Although the foregoing data-base outline allows for multidisciplinary input, it tends to be designed primarily for a physician's history and physical examination. Nurses can add to this data base through the nursing history or the initial patient interview.

Problem List

The second component, the problem list, is a carefully managed listing of problems that the professionals believe to require intervention. This list becomes the index to the chart. Each problem is numbered and is subsequently always referred to by that number. Specific rules for what constitutes a problem and how one is added or deleted are a necessary part of this procedure. This list provides an overview of the patient's health status.

Initial Plan

The initial plan for any episode of care is the first entry on the multidisciplinary progress notes. The plan should include three elements: further data-gathering, therapeutic orders, and client education instructions.

Progress Notes

The progress notes continue in what is referred to as the "SOAP" format:

SUBJECTIVE: What the patient says or reports about the problem.

OBJECTIVE: What the professional directly observes regarding clinical or behavioral manifestations.

ASSESSMENT: What the professional concludes relative to the response of the patient to treatment and/or care. (This is the evaluative aspect of the SOAP note.)

PLAN: What the professional intends to do or to have done relative to the problem.[6]

As the episode of care continues, each professional enters any pertinent information by problem number in the SOAP format. The last progress note entry is referred to as a discharge summary. Again, in SOAP format, all the current problems are summarized. This summary provides the background for a problem list during subsequent episodes of care. An example of problem-oriented documentation is shown in Fig. 3.1. The advantages of this problem-oriented system are several. It focuses everyone's attention on the client's problems; it facilitates multidisciplinary audit; it centralizes information; and it provides a classification and coding system that all disciplines must consistently utilize. Some possible disadvantages of this system are that each professional must find and read through several SOAP notes to determine the current status of the client, and there is some redundancy from one SOAP note to the next. This becomes particularly evident in an acute-care setting. There is also a logistical disadvantage in the tracing of many problems with many numbers throughout the progress notes. In actual practice, there is a tendency for one or two problems to be traced, leaving the remainder to haphazard follow-up.

Outcome-Oriented

An outcome-oriented system of documentation was originally designed for organizing the nursing process in a functional written form. Its focus is on the client's goals or outcomes and all recording is done with reference to the client's current status measured against the desired outcome as a decision standard. Outcome-oriented charting is also designed to be compatible with client-outcome auditing procedures. "The major components of outcome-oriented charting are: Data base (nursing history), problem identification (usual and unusual), desired client outcomes (clinical and behavioral, short-term objectives), deadlines for evaluation and documentation, nursing orders, outcome documentation (progress notes), and standards for discharge or maintenance (long-term objectives)."[6]

Data Base

A data base is a collection of relevant facts which describe a client's status. For each episode of care, an updated compilation of baseline data (or relevant facts) is required in order to make inferences leading to nursing diagnoses. The organizing scheme for a data-collection guide should be based upon a conceptual framework which provides the cues for gathering the facts.

Problem Identification

A problem or nursing diagnosis is a testable conclusion or judgment stating the client's variance from a desired health standard and the reason for the variance. Nursing diagnoses as problems can take two forms, "usual" and "unusual." "Usual problems are difficulties or concerns anticipated for most patients with a given diagnosis (medical or nursing)..."[6] Unique or unpredictable difficulties or concerns experienced by a client are considered unusual. "Problem statements are usually documented on the care plan"[6] which becomes a part of the legal client record. A nursing diagnosis may reflect the conclusion that there is no variance from a desired health standard.

80

Figure 3.1
Example of Problem-Oriented Documentation

Date	No.	Inactive/Resolved Problems	Date Resolved
10/21	1	COPD c̄ Cor Pulmonale	
10/21	2	SOB c̄ Orthopnea	
10/21	3	Edema of feet & ascites	
10/21	4	Chest pain	
10/21	5	Chronic depression	
10/21	6	Osteoporosis — unknown etiology	
10/21	7	Compression Fx T7-T8	1968
10/21	1	COPD c̄ Cor Pulmonale — Further Tests: Monitor exertion-fatigue ratio; Monitor food & fluid intake. Treatment: Regulate activity; Six small feedings/day; Spread fluid intake over 24° period. Teaching: Quiet environment; Relationship of activity to fatigue; Potential life style alteration & planning.	
10/21	2	SOB c̄ Orthopnea — See above.	
10/21	3	Edema & Ascites — Further Tests: Monitor degree q̄ shift.	

Date	#	Diagnosis	
			Treatment: Foot cradle; skin care.
			Teaching: Cause of edema & how prevented; Pt. manage own fluid intake before discharge.
10/21	4	Chest Pain	Further Tests: Monitor absence or presence of chest pain q̄ shift.
			Treatment: Limit activity; stay c̄ pt. when in pain.
10/21	5	Chronic Depression	Further Tests: Interview re: causes for onset & freq. of episodes of depression.
			Treatment: Active listening.
			Teaching: Direct toward "insight".
10/21	6	Osteoporosis	Further Tests: Monitor for absence or presence of deep bone pain; Report any flank pain.
			Treatment: ∅
			Teaching: Explain decalcification & relationship to decrease & dietary treatment. A. Riley, RN

Figure 3.1 *(cont.)*

Example of Problem-Oriented Documentation*

Date	No.	Problem	Progress Notes
10/22	2	SOB c̄ Orthopnea	S: "I had to sit up all last night. "States couldn't complete bath s resting.[11]
			O: Rapid respirations, expiratory wheeze & cyanotic nailbed in sitting position.
			A: Problem essentially the same as on admission.
			P: Continue initial plan. A. Riley, RN
10/23	3	Edema & Ascites	S: "I feel like I'm 6 months pregnant" — says he has to urinate frequently.
			O: Abdomen distended, firm & tender to touch. Ankles 2° pitting edema. No edema of legs & arms.
			A: Beginning to respond to diuretic treatment.
			P: Continue initial plan. A. Riley, RN

Date	No.	Problem	Progress Notes
11/20	2	SOB c̄ Orthopnea	S: Verbalizes satisfaction c̄ own ability to pace ADL. States he is on 6-month medical leave from work. Wife states she has converted downstairs den into bedroom to minimize stair climbing.
			O: Past week has done all own care without fatigue & s̄ episodes of SOB. Has demonstrated ability to recognize the problem & make realistic plans for home & job.
			A: Responding satisfactorily to prescribed plan of care.
			P: Referral to home health agency to evaluate adaptation to home environment. B. Weatherby, RN

*From Mayers, Norby and Watson: Quality Assurance for Patient Care: Nursing Perspectives, 1977, pp. 151, 153-155. Courtesy of Appleton-Century-Crofts, Publishers.

Desired Client Outcomes

Desirable outcomes are written phrases describing what client behavior/s and clinical manifestation/s will reflect the fact that the problem is satisfactorily resolved or is in process of being resolved. The formulation of desired outcomes is the predictive element of the nursing process. These are the standards for continual assessment and evaluation of the client's status.

Deadlines for Evaluation and Documentation

Inherent in the expected outcome phrases are those time frames for ongoing assessment, outcome achievement, and documentation. Desired outcomes with their deadlines are in essence behavioral objectives. Each objective contains an action verb, content, and a performance standard. An example might be "Ambulates with crutches, using a three-point gait by four days prior to discharge." Forming objectives in the planning process enables one to observe, measure, and describe desired changes.[7,8]

Nursing Orders

The prescription element of the nursing process is reflected in what is referred to as nursing orders. These are the interventions or methodologies (defensible alternatives) for achieving desired outcomes.

Outcome Documentation

Although all the elements of the nursing process are documented, the "outcome documentation" element specifically refers to the written descriptions and evaluative recordings of the nurse's perceptions of the client's status. These recordings refer to the desired outcomes as standards for comparison and evaluative judgments. This is the feedback loop of the nursing process. The expected outcome serves as a yardstick against which to measure progress or achievement.

Standards for Discharge or Maintenance

Standards for discharge or maintenance are formulated, using the same rules as for desired outcomes. These discharge standards, however, refer to those clinical and behavioral expectations that should have been achieved by the completion of a given episode of care.

A basic advantage of outcome-oriented documentation is that it is consistent with outcome auditing, thus reinforcing both the nursing process and its concurrent and retrospective auditing mechanisms. It can easily be used with both source-oriented and problem-oriented methods of organizing data. Because of its focus on outcome, it validates the client's response, thereby acting as a check for nursing actions. Disadvantages, as with any comprehensive documentation system, are that it requires a refocus of thinking, a shift from placing emphasis on what the nurse does to an emphasis on the client's response to what the nurse does. This shift in focus is energy-consuming and requires support and reinforcement during learning phases. For complicated clients, this method of documentation results in voluminous amounts of information which must be organized according to specific rules and regulations. An example of outcome documentation is shown in Fig. 3.2. This client is a 55-year-old man whose admitting diagnosis is chronic obstructive pulmonary disease.

COMPONENTS OF A COMPREHENSIVE DOCUMENTATION SYSTEM

Whichever major method of documentation is adopted, each of the three previously described methods requires the use of specific forms to insure comprehensive documentation.

Care Plans

Care-plan forms are probably the best-known components of any client-centered documentation system. All professional disciplines require documentation of the thought process unique to its function. Nursing functions are documented through what is commonly called the patient care plan. The operational parts of a care plan normally include client problems, long- and short-term goals, and nursing interventions. The plan can be organized in a variety of ways as long as it is comprehensive and current. It documents the quality of the analytic process used in providing client care. This, then, enables colleagues to criticize and consult retrospectively and concurrently about a given client's plan of care. The growing trend in nursing for the care plan to become a part of the client's permanent record is a good development. Care plans for day-to-day operational purposes should be located where they are most accessible to the care-givers. They may be found at the bedside, on clip boards, in binders, in a cardex, on rands, in rolladex files, in file boxes, or in computer memory banks. An example of a care-plan format is shown in Fig. 3.3. For a care plan with written entries, refer to Fig. 3.2.

An important element of a care-planning system is the "standard care plan." This is a care plan developed and prewritten for clients who experience predictable or "usual" problems. These plans contain the basic, the usually anticipated, nursing-care information. They make clear, in written form, those care requirements that may otherwise be left to chance.[9] "Because prewritten standard care plans are applicable to large numbers of patients, they eliminate the need to handwrite large quantities of repetitive

Figure 3.2

Example of Outcome-Oriented Documentation†

Care Plan

Nursing's Criteria for Discharge or Maintenance: 1) See Standard Care Plan for COPD 2) Correctly reiterate medication regimen & potential side effects 3) Wife to correctly plan week's Lo Na menu 4) Pt. & wife verbalize realistic plans for home & social activities 5) Verbalize signs & symptoms & appropriate action to take.

DISCHARGE PLANNING: Notify HHA for follow-up to assess pt's. adaptation to home environment. (Referral made 11/1, AW, RN)

Date	Problems	Expected Outcomes	Deadlines	Nursing Orders
10/21	See Standard Care Plan for COPD			
10/21	1. Unrelieved abdominal pain & nausea due to K level at 3.2 m Eq	1. no c/o abdominal pain electrolytes within normal limits	√ daily p.m. shift	1. a. Check daily electrolyte level. b. Call M.D. & notify of any abnormal "lytes" level. c. Question medical order of Lasix 80 mg. b.i.d. s̄ K Cl replacement.

B. Murray, R.N.

Age: 55 Date Admitted: 10-21-74 Diagnosis: Chronic Obstructive Pulmonary Disease c̄ Cor Pulmonale Ht. 5'5"
Wt. 154 Date of Surgery: — Surgery: — Religion: Protestant Notify in Case of Emergency: Mrs. P.
Telephone: (415) 000-000 Name: P., Jack Doctor: Wells Room No. 5515-C

Nurses Notes

Date & Time	Nurses Notes
10/21 3:00 P.M.	Complains of constant abdominal cramping and sensation of pressure and nausea. Potassium remains elevated. Is too fatigued to begin teaching program. A. Riley, RN
10/22 2:30 P.M.	Abdominal cramping & nausea persists. Abdomen tender to touch. Potassium elevated. No teaching yet. A. Riley, RN
10/22 9:30 P.M.	Fifteen minutes spent c̄ wife determining her response to pt's. illness. Verbalizes concern over pt's. immediate health status & fears he may not return to work. S. Andrews, RN
10/23 11:00 A.M.	States that cramping is less severe & only intermittent. Abdomen is still tender. Only one episode of nausea this A.M. B. Brown, RN
10/23 8:30 P.M.	Wife reiterated fears & concerns & unable to respond to problem-solving attempts. R. Johnson, RN

Many days elapse with charting occurring similar to that illustrated above, except that both flow sheet and narrative show possible progress for this patient. Following is an example of the nurses' discharge note on 11/20.

Date & Time	Nurses Notes
11/20 1:00 P.M.	Discharge summary: Past two weeks has correctly done own IPPB using same equipment to be used at home. Has done correct self-medication past week in hospital & today correctly reiterated each Rx, why he's taking it, the side effects of each and appropriate action to take. Correctly stated his potential complications & what to do if S/S arise. During past week he & his wife have calmly discussed specific plans for: moving bedroom downstairs; pacing ADL; revising eating pattern to frequent small meals; and plans to have friends in & out to lodge activities. Wife submitted one week's Lo Na menu. Referred to Home Health agency made on 11/1. First home visit to be made within one week. A. Riley, RN

†From Mayers, Norby and Watson: Quality Assurance for Patient Care, Nursing Perspectives, 1977, pp 39, 40. Courtesy of Appleton-Century-Crofts, Publishers.

88

Figure 3.3
Example of a Care-Plan Format

CARE PLAN

STANDARDS FOR DISCHARGE OR MAINTENANCE: _____

DATE	PROBLEMS	EXPECTED OUTCOMES	DEADLINES	NURSING ORDERS	COMPLETED

information."[9] (In chapter 2, Fig. 2.1 gives an example of a standard care plan.)

Narratives

Narratives are written descriptions relating the details of the nursing process—assessment, intervention, client response, and evaluation. Narrative notes can be structured and nonstructured. In traditional source-oriented charting, narrative notes (nurses' notes) are generally less structured in format, with entries governed by charting policy and procedure. Problem-oriented narratives are structured according to the SOAP format. Outcome-oriented narratives are more structured, with prescribed entries dictated by expected outcomes and deadlines. Figs. 3.4, 3.5, and 3.6 show examples of narratives, each reflecting a different documentation method.

Flow Sheets

Flow sheets are graphic displays designed in horizontal and vertical columns to accommodate multiple information variables across time. Familiar to all nurses are flow sheets such as the TPR graphic, the intake and output record, or the anticoagulant record. Flow sheets can be used with any of the three major documentation methods. They can be designed with predetermined variables that relate to specific, commonly-occurring situations, such as hemodynamic monitoring. Or they can allow for individualized variables or clinical parameters to be written in for monitoring purposes. Fig. 3.7 shows a flow sheet with predetermined variables; Fig. 3.8 shows one with individualized variables and entries.

Another variation of a flow sheet which can be predetermined and individualized suggests variables derived from standard care plans or audit criteria. Figs. 3.9 and 3.10 show examples of a care plan with an associated predetermined flow sheet for clients experiencing chronic obstructive pulmonary disease. It will be noticed that the expected outcomes from the care plan have been abbreviated into clinical parameters as guides for assessment and documentation.

Flow sheets may be interpreted as shorthand versions of narratives. They are particularly valuable for situations involving rapidly changing values relative to clinical parameters such as those in intensive-care settings. The time involved in setting up a flow sheet is short in contrast to the time involved in writing, assembling, and retrieving information from various parts of a chart. It is important to strike a balance between an exhaustive list of variables and a "compulsive preoccupation with the precision of a single variable, which, if interpreted by itself, could be very misleading."[4]

The authors have observed that it is sometimes difficult to document detailed psycho-social or learning responses of clients within the limited

Figure 3.4
A Nonstructured Narrative Note

DATE	NURSE'S NOTES
1/29 11 A.M.	Resting quietly on right side. No obvious shortness of breath during the past hour. Slight pitting of ankles this morning following ambulation. A. Johnson, R.N.

This is a patient whose medical diagnosis is congestive heart failure. The nurse's note refers to only one element of a larger spectrum of information about the client.

Figure 3.5
A Problem-Oriented Narrative Note

DATE	NO.	PROBLEM	PROGRESS NOTES
1/29 11 A.M.	5	Ankle Edema	S "My feet feel so puffy and heavy." O Pitting Edema noted about both ankles. A Due to decreased circulation to extremities. P Keep both legs elevated; continue diuretic therapy as ordered; Continue 2 Gm. Na. diet; Encourage patient to dorsiflex feet."[10] A. Johnson, R.N.

This is a patient whose medical diagnosis is congestive heart failure. The nurse's note refers to only one problem from the problem list.

space provided on flow sheets. Flow sheets are good examples of the assembling, coding, and classification elements of communication presented at the beginning of this chapter.

Figure 3.6
An Outcome-Oriented Narrative Note

DATE	PROGRESS NOTES
11/29	1+ pitting edema of both ankles after sitting in chair with feet elevated for twenty minutes. Weight 182 pounds at 7 a.m. Remains 4 pounds above normal.
	Urinary output of 200 cc. since 7 A.M.
	A. Johnson, R.N.

This is a client whose medical diagnosis is congestive heart failure. The notes respond to care-plan outcomes for one "usual" problem. The desired outcomes are:

- No ankle edema   √ daily A.M.
- Body weight at pre-congestive episode
- Urinary output at least 240 cc/shift

Referrals

A referral is the act of sending or directing specific information or instructions for purposes of further interventions and decisions. A referral is one example of external communication, sending information from one system to another. A referral is normally initiated when one individual, group, or system lacks the expertise or resources to solve one or more aspects of a situation. Thus, the referral represents partial or complete closure of responsibility on the part of one care provider and transmits the information necessary for another to assume responsibility.

Any referral documentation should include the following categories of information:

- reasons for referral
- demographic client data
- continuing problems
- general level of adaptation
- specific nursing, medical, or other orders
- client's goals (health situation, life, level of function)
- resources available to client
- feedback route to referring person or agency

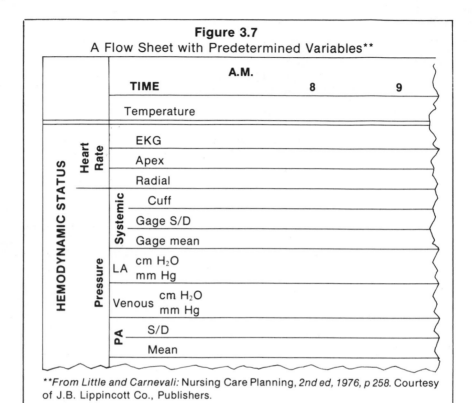

Figure 3.7
A Flow Sheet with Predetermined Variables**

		A.M.		
	TIME		8	9
	Temperature			

HEMODYNAMIC STATUS

Heart Rate
- EKG
- Apex
- Radial

Pressure — Systemic
- Cuff
- Gage S/D
- Gage mean

LA
- cm H$_2$O
- mm Hg

Venous
- cm H$_2$O
- mm Hg

PA
- S/D
- Mean

**From Little and Carnevali: Nursing Care Planning, *2nd ed, 1976, p 258.* Courtesy of J.B. Lippincott Co., Publishers.

The referral document itself may take various forms. Again, these forms may be structured on nonstructured. Specific headings, topics, and categories for forms can be developed through the cooperative efforts of referring groups. Adjuncts to a referral which are frequently helpful are care plans and discharge summaries.

A variation of a referral form is a transfer form. The basic difference is that a transfer normally occurs between units within an organization (lateral communication). In most instances, the same kinds of information are required for transfer as for referral. Frequently the information is already available through the client's chart and care plan. Thus, a separate transfer form may not be required. However, some units or groups that frequently transfer clients from one to another have developed transfer forms. The primary purpose in both referral and transfer documentation is to minimize time lost in understanding the client situation and to maximize the quality of services required to meet the client's goals, thereby insuring continuity of care.

Figure 3.8
A Flow Sheet with Individualized Variables and Entries‡

FLOW SHEET

Diabetics (Dx 4/9)

Variables	Time					
	4/10	4/11	4/12	4/13	4/14	4/15
Hypoglycemic Episodes	X2	X1	0	0	0	0
Weight	115	112	111	111	111	110
Insulin techniques	by RN	LP & gf watching steps	LP meas. RN inj.	LP meas. accurately & inj. JP watch	JP meas. LP inj.	JP meas. & inj. 1x LP meas. & inj. 1x
Urine testing	RN	RN explain (+ written info) & show LP/JP	LP explaining & demon. to RN	LP explaining to JP & testing	JP explaining & testing	LP Testing on own
Urine Sug/Kit	4+/4+	2+/0	0/0	tr/0	tr/0	0/0
Ambulation	0	5' x 2	30' x 2	30' x 3	ad lib	ad lib
Diet Food Composition	/	Explored: Understanding	RN identifies Hi COH, Fat & Prot. food on tray	Lack of interest	List of food composition given	Identified COH Fat Prot comp. of food on tray x3

Figure 3.8 *(cont.)*
A Flow Sheet with Individualized Variables and Entries‡

FLOW SHEET

Diabetics (Dx 4/9)

Time

Variables						
Rx diet	/	/	/	Explored implications LP angry JP worried	Cont. discussion of implications for	Showed MD Rx diet
Exchange diet	/	/	/	/	How to get control by knowing exchange system	Planned menus X3 days built on family patterns & lists. LP/JP
Relationship of blood sugar to life events	0 Understanding	LP Angry JP interested	Explored that understanding control c LP	Asked LP to relate usual phys act to BS	LP Emot. stresses & B sugar	Illness & B sugar

‡From Little and Carnevali: Nursing Care Planning, 2nd ed, 1976, p 262. Courtesy of J.B. Lippincott, Co., Publishers.

Figure 3.9

A Standard Care Plan for Chronic Obstructive Pulmonary Disease*

Standards for Discharge or Maintenance: (1) Verbalize understanding of and willingness to follow MDs discharge medical regime; (2) Verbalize realistic plans for home care; (3) Demonstrate correct use of breathing apparatus, pulmonary exercise regimen; (4) Reiterate a plan for self-pacing of activities in home environment; (5) Correctly administer own medications X 4 days before discharge.

DISCHARGE PLANNING: Referral to Respiratory Care Nurse for home evaluation and adjustment.

Date	Usual Problems	Expected Outcomes	Deadlines	Nursing Orders
	1. SOB, dyspnea.	1. Display minimal to no SOB	√ q̄ 8 hr	1. A. Elevate head of bed. B. Teach breathing techniques (pursed lips). C. Bedrest — minimize activity. D. Monitor O_2 to avoid O_2 toxicity.
	2. Chronic fatigue due to decreased circulating O_2.	2. A. Verbalize less fatigue. B. Pulse ↓ 100 per minute. C. Eat all meals and assist c̄ care s̄ undue fatigue.	√ q̄ 8 hr	2. A. Keep frequently used items within easy reach. B. Arrange schedule to allow maximum rest. C. 6 small feedings may be helpful. D. Bedside commode.
	3. Apprehension and anxiety due to SOB.	3. A. Remain calm — show optimism. B. Sleep all night.	√ daily A.M.	3. A. Staff remains calm and unhurried when in room. B. Provide opportunity for pt to verbalize fears.

Figure 3.9 (cont.)

A Standard Care Plan for Chronic Obstructive Pulmonary Disease*

Date	Usual Problems	Expected Outcomes	Deadlines	Nursing Orders
	4. Potential respiratory failure due to hypoxia and hypercapnea.	4. A. Display adequate ventilation. B. Asymptomatic of cyanosis or CO_2 narcosis.	√ q̄ 8 hr	4. A. Obtain order for arterial blood gases. B. Assess ABG results and inform MD. C. Have assistive ventilation equipment nearby. D. Have trach equipment in room for emergency.
	5. Potential electrolyte imbalance (respiratory acidosis).	5. A. Show no sign of impending acidosis. B. Lucid and oriented to reality.	√ q̄ 8 hr	5. A. Obtain order for electrolytes to be drawn. B. Evaluate above lab values. C. Observe for signs of restlessness, confusion, tachycardia or bradycardia, diaphoresis, headache, tremors or muscle flaccidity.
	6. Potential respiratory infection.	6. A. Lungs sound clear. B. Temp ↓ 100F. C. Pulse ↓ 100 per min. D. Sputum cultures negative.	√ q̄ 8 hr	6. A. Obtain order for suction PRN. B. Evaluate color and consistency of sputum. C. Obtain order for sputum culture. D. Instruct on coughing technique. E. Encourage to cough at least q̄ 1 hr.
	7. Potential CHF due to increased work load of heart.	7. A. Lungs sound clear. B. BP 140/90. C. No presence of edema in extremities.	√ q̄ 8 hr	7. A. Monitor I and 0 carefully. B. Obtain order for anti-emboli stockings. C. Observe for signs of impending CHF.

Problem	Expected Outcomes	Date	Nursing Orders
	ties or jugular venous distention. D. Heart rate within normal limits. E. Has no cardiac arrhythmias.		D. Obtain order (or standing order) for rotating tourniquets in emergency.
8. Potential osteoporosis due to decalcification.	8. Verbalize no increase of deep bone pain.	√ daily A.M.	8. Monitor presence or absence of deep bone or flank pain.
9. Potential peptic ulcer due to increased gastric secretions and psychopathology.	9. No evidence of gastric distress, hematemesis, abdominal soreness, no blood in stools.	√ q̄ 8 hr	9. A. Monitor abdominal pain q̄ shift. B. Palpate abdomen q̄ shift. C. Observe any emesis for blood. D. Check stool for occult blood q̄ day if evidence of gastric distress.
10. Concern for home management.	10. Verbalizes: A. realistic arrangement for IPPB or nebulizer at home. B. understanding of medical and dietary regimen.	A. √ daily P.M. / B. 24 hours prior to discharge	10. A. Respiratory therapist or RN instruct pt on IPPB if to be used at home. B. Teach about medicine to be used at home and medical regimen. C. Dietician instruct on diet — RN follow-up prior to discharge.
11. Potential concern over financial and occupational implication due to chronic disabling condition.	11. Verbalize realistic plans for finances and job.	√ By discharge / √ q̄ week P.M.	11. One nurse problem solve c̄ pt daily and coordinate referral to social services or home care.

*Adapted from Mayers, Watson and Norby: Quality Assurance for Patient Care, Nursing Perspectives, 1977, pp 137, 138. Courtesy of Appleton-Century-Crofts, Publishers.

Figure 3.10

A Flow Sheet for Chronic Obstructive Pulmonary Disease†

Clinical Parameters		DATES				
		10/21	10/22	10/23	10/24	10/25
SOB Activity/Fatigue	AM	11:00 Fatigue c̄ breathing	10:00 Constant fatigue	10:00 Rested s̄ activity	9:00 Limited ADL s̄ SOB	9:00 Limited s̄ SOB
	PM	7:00 Same	8:00 Same	8:00 Same	7:00 Same	7:00 Same
	NOC	1:00 Orthopnea	2:00 Orthopnea	Sleeps in high Fowler	Sleeps in high Fowler	Sleeps in high Fowler
Anxiety Level	PM	Anxious 7:00 calls freq.	Anxious 8:00 calls often	Fewer calls 8:00 less anxious	Anxious 8:15 at times	Anxious 7:00 at times
Cyanosis: (presence or absence)	AM	Presence nailbeds	Presence nailbeds	Presence nailbeds	Presence nailbeds	Presence nailbeds
	PM	7:00 Same	8:00 Same	8:00 Same	7:00 Same	7:00 Same
	NOC	1:00 Same	2:00 Same	2:00 Same	2:00 Same	2:30 Same
Headache: (presence or absence)	AM	11:00 Present	10:00 Present	10:00 None	9:00 None	9:00 None
	PM	7:00 Same	8:00 Same	8:00 None	7:00 None	7:00 None
	NOC	1:00 Same	1:00 Same	1:30 None	2:00 None	2:30 None

Assessment	Shift					
Mentation/ Orientation/ Sleep	AM	9:00 Oriented but slow mentation	10:00 Same	Oriented alert	Oriented alert	9:00 Same
Lung Sounds	AM	Moist Rales	Moist Rales	Moist Rales	Faint Rales	Faint Rales
	PM	7:00 Same	8:00 Same	8:00 Same	7:00 Same	7:00 Same
	NOC	2:00 Same	2:00 Same	1:30 Same	4:00 Same	2:30 Same
Edema: (° of pitting-ankle)	AM	11:00 3°	10:00 3°	10:00 2°	9:00 2°	9:00 2°
	PM	7:00 3°	10:00 3°	8:00 2°	8:00 2°	7:00 2°
	NOC	2:00 3°	2:00 3°	1:30 2°	4:00 2°	2:30 2°
Deep Bone Pain	AM	9:00 on arising	—	—	—	—
Learning Response (pt. and spouse)	AM	See narrative notes				
	PM	See narrative notes				
Gastric Distress/ Abd. Soreness/ Hematemesis	AM	See narrative notes				
	PM	See narrative notes				
	NOC	See narrative notes				
SIGNATURE:	AM	S. Andrews RN	E. Johnson RN			
SIGNATURE:	PM	K. Tyler RN				
SIGNATURE:	NOC	A. Riley RN				

†From Mayers, Norby and Watson: Quality Assurance for Patient Care, Nursing Perspectives, 1977, p 139. Courtesy of Appleton-Century-Crofts, Publishers.

DOCUMENTING THE
ASSESSMENT PROCESS

Two client situations are presented to illustrate how theories are put to use in a practical way. The interactive/affiliative system of man and its theories are used as a basis for formulating standards, for developing data-collection guides and for arriving at a nursing diagnosis. The two clients are Janice and Mrs. Ellison who were introduced in chapter 2. In this chapter a documentation form that aids in theory-based asessment is used. The form has preprinted standards for the interactive/affiliative system. It has check ($\checkmark$) boxes for the inference and validation steps, and a blank column for handwriting a nursing diagnosis for each standard. The form also has preprinted questions, observations, and examinations to assist the nurse in obtaining theory-related data from the client. The client data lead one to make decisions relative to the standards.

The questions as shown on the assessment guide represent only one system of man and do not represent all the questions one may wish to include for a complete nursing history. The assessment form as shown is designed to guide one through the phases of assessment. This form, or a variation of it, can become part of the chart, thereby reducing the necessity to summarize or rewrite information.

Scenario 1

Table 3.1 (p. 125) shows an assessment guide for Janice, the client described in scenario 1.

Documenting the Planning Process

The most common method of documenting the planning phase of the nursing process is the care plan. To illustrate this phase, a care plan (Fig. 3.11) is based on the diagnoses (deductions) formulated in scenario 1 and as shown in the last column of the nursing assessment guide. Following the care plan, the three methods of charting are illustrated. The same series of documentation steps are illustrated for Mrs. Allison in scenario 2.

Methods of Charting

Source-Oriented—The following documentation illustrates source-oriented nurses' notes relative to scenario 1, Janice. The notations assume that the nursing history and the care plan are not part of the permanent record. Therefore the notations summarize much of what has already been illustrated earlier in this chapter. (See p. 103)

Figure 3.11

Care Plan, Scenario One, Janice

STANDARDS FOR DISCHARGE OR MAINTENANCE: *Makes a decision regarding future of pregnancy by 11/2.*

DATE	PROBLEMS	EXPECTED OUTCOMES	DEADLINES	NURSING ORDERS	COMPLETED
10/12	2. Constant insecurity due to conflict between self-expectations, achievements, and whether or not to terminate pregnancy.	2. Verbalizes pros and cons of terminating pregnancy. Verbalizes feelings of decreased tension. Makes a decision regarding future of pregnancy.	√ q̄ visit 3 weeks (Nov 2)	2a. Home or clinic visit 2 times weekly. b. Use reflective listening at each visit. c. Explore alternatives and consequences with her. d. Provide resources available in community depending upon decision client makes. (Abortion services or prenatal services)	

Figure 3.11 *(cont.)*
Care Plan, Scenario One, Janice

STANDARDS FOR DISCHARGE OR MAINTENANCE: *Makes a decision regarding future of pregnancy by 11/2.*

DATE	PROBLEMS	EXPECTED OUTCOMES	DEADLINES	NURSING ORDERS	COMPLETED
10/12	3. Sudden role ambivalency due to unplanned pregnancy.	3. Discusses life goals and role possibilities.	√ q̄ visit	3. See #1	
	4. Uncertainty due to change in future role and establishing a relationship with another man.	4. Expresses feelings about prior and future relationships with men.	√ q̄ visit	4. See 1B Suggest perusing bookstores for current literature on "male-female" relationships. A. Johnson, R.N.	

This care plan represents only the interactive/affiliative assessment of Janice. It is assumed that at least one problem from another system of man has been diagnosed and listed as problem number 1.

DATE	NURSE'S NOTES (Source-Oriented)
10/12	*Home Visit:* Client is a 29-year-old female, 2½ months pregnant. Articulate, communicative, and seemingly at ease with interviewer. Expresses confusion and depression over this unplanned pregnancy, especially because ex-boyfriend has left her. Her primary concern at this time is to come to a decision as to whether or not to terminate the pregnancy. Other concerns, although not immediate, are related to ambivalence over future role, career, and self-identity as a woman, and relationships with men in the future. Her personal support systems are her sister, who lives nearby, and her mother, who lives in another state. She works as a section manager in a personnel department and expresses satisfaction with both her job and work relationships. Expresses dissatisfaction with lack of her ability to maintain social-group relationships outside of work. Has a history of feeling satisfied with accomplishments and says that she usually feels in control of situations, yet also says life tends to happen by accident. Has nearly completed her college degree. Enjoys reading and traveling, but says that she now is "frittering" away her leisure time. Assumes many roles: career girl, student, boss, sister and says: "I'm already beginning to feel like a mother." Expresses some strong feelings about loss of ex-boyfriend but has decided against contacting him. Expresses a desire to continue discussing her situation with nurse. *Problems Identified:* 1. Constant insecurity conflict between self-expectations and achievements and whether or not to terminate pregnancy. 2. Sudden role ambivalency due to unplanned pregnancy. 3. Uncertainty due to change in future role and establishing a relationship with another man. *Objectives:* Janice will make a decision regarding the future of her pregnancy by 11/2.

104

Plan:

Visit 2x per week for 3 weeks; assist Janice through reflective listening, exploring consequences of alternatives, and providing community resources as decision process unfolds;

Suggest she read current literature on male-female relationships.

A. Johnson, R.N.

INTERIM NOTE

10/26   *Home Visit:*

At this time, Janice says she has decided to have an abortion. Double-checking with her regarding her feelings and her decision process results in the conclusion that, all things considered, she is satisfied with this decision. States she has discussed decision with sister and has decided not to tell mother of entire situation. Says that she personally discussed her feelings with ex-boyfriend and he concurs with her decision. She wept when talking about her decision, yet was also able to laugh and smile when thinking about the future. Has selected two books but has not started reading them yet — too preoccupied with what to do. Asked for referral to an abortion clinic. Given information and phone numbers of three clinics in area. Encouraged her to call nurse if any problems in making contact or appointments with clinic. Discussed with her what she can expect from the clinic services and how she can be assertive enough that her physical and emotional needs are met. Asked Janice whether or not she wishes nurse to continue to visit. She stated that she is confident she can follow through independently now that she has made her decision. She will call nurse, however, if unforeseen problems develop. Nurse agrees to call in one month to see how things are going before closing to service.

A. Johnson, R.N.

DISCHARGE NOTE

11/26   *Telephone Call:*

Janice reports that her experience at the abortion clinic was satisfactory in all respects. Her pregnancy was terminated on 11/5 and she was assisted by a counselor throughout the entire experience. She says she knows that she has many unresolved feelings about the abortion and will see the counselor a few more times until she feels more stable. When asked if she has thought about her life goals, career, and relationships with men, she says that her first concern is to think through "being myself" rather than focusing on men or life goals right now.

Closed to service.

A. Johnson, R.N.

In the event that the nursing history (assessment guide) and care plan are part of the permanent record, a brief notation can substitute for all the previous progress notes. The initial entry might have been abbreviated to:

Client is 29-year-old female, 2½ months pregnant Articulate, communicative, and seems at ease with the interviewer. See nursing history and care plan.

A. Johnson, R.N.

Problem-Oriented—The following chart illustrates problem-oriented documentation relative to scenario 1. The data base is documented in the nursing assessment guide for Janice shown in Table 3.1, page 21. The other components of problem-oriented charting are problem list, initial plan, progress notes, and discharge summary.

PROBLEM LIST

DATE	ACTIVE PROBLEMS	INACTIVE PROBLEMS
10/12 1.	Pregnancy, 2½ months Gestation H. Wells, M.D. 10/26 3 mos. gestation 11/26 resolved	
10/12 2.	Constant insecurity due to conflict between self-expectations and achievements and whether or not to terminate pregnancy. 10/26 resolved	

PROBLEM LIST (cont.)

10/12 *3.*	Sudden role ambivalency due to unplanned pregnancy (secondary to problem 2). 10/26 2 constant insecurity	
10/12 *4.*	Uncertainty due to change in future role and establishing relationship with another man. 11/26 resolved	

INITIAL PLAN

1. Pregnancy, 2½ months gestation.

Diagnostic Plans	CBC, and blood type, blood glucose.
Therapeutic Plans	Multivitamins with calcium.
Patient-Education Plans	Patient given diet instructions. Recommended 18-22 lb. overall weight gain. Instructed if bleeding or cramping occurs call physician immediately. Return visit in one month.

                H. Wells, M.D.

2. Constant insecurity due to conflict between self-expectations and achievements and whether or not to terminate pregnancy.

Diagnostic Plans	Determine feelings and realities regarding pregnancy.
Therapeutic Plans	Reflective listening and exploration of alternatives and their consequences. Home visits 2x weekly for 3 weeks.
Patient-Education Plans	Provide information regarding community resources depending upon decision process (abortion services or prenatal services).

3. Sudden role ambivalency due to unplanned pregnancy (see 2).

4. Uncertainty due to change in future role and establishing a relationship with another man.

Diagnostic Plans	Identify feelings about prior and future relationships with men.
Therapeutic Plans	Reflective listening.
Patient-Education Plans	Suggest she read current literature on "male-female relationships."
	A. Johnson, R.N.

PROGRESS NOTES

DATE	NO.	PROBLEM	PROGRESS NOTES
INTERIM 10/26	1	Pregnancy, 2 mos. gestation	S — Says physically feeling ok. Has gained 2 lbs in last mo. Did not buy multi-vitamins nor get blood work done.
			O — No laboratory data in chart. Weight 124 lbs.
			A — Has decided for self not to initiate prenatal care at this time.
			P — See problem 2.
			H. Wells, M.D.
10/26	2	Constant insecurity	S — States she has decided to have an abortion; states she is satisfied with this decision.
			O — Wept when talking about decision, yet able to laugh and smile when thinking about future.
			A — Is satisfied with decision.
		Action*	Referred to 3 abortion clinic services. Reviewed what to expect from services and rights she can assume — physical, emotional. Encouraged to call nurse if any problems develop.

| | | | P — Phone in one month before closing to service. |
| | | | A. Johnson, R.N. |

Action — *This type of notation is not part of the SOAP format. However, the POMR system allows for the documentation of other information as needed. Thus an action step has been included. Problem 3 was not SOAPed because it was classified as secondary to problem 2. There would not, therefore, be any additional information to document because problem 2 was resolved on this date. Problem 4 was not included on the progress notes (SOAPed) because no information was gathered relative to this problem on the visit of 10/26.*

DATE	NO.	PROBLEM	PROGRESS NOTES
		DISCHARGE SUMMARY	
11/26	1	Pregnancy	S — States abortion completed on 11/5. Experience was satisfactory. Is following up with counselor.
11/26	2	Constant insecurity	Resolved
11/26	3	Sudden role ambivalency	Resolved
11/26	4	Uncertainty due to change in future role and establishing a relationship with another man	S — States that she wants to focus on "being myself, rather than on relationships with men or life goals."
			O — _____
			A — Exploring current perception of self and role.
			P — Closed to service.
			A. Johnson, R.N.

The POMR documentation for Janice did not require the use of a flow sheet. There were only a few variables and these did not fluctuate greatly within a short period of time.

Outcome-Oriented —Outcome-oriented charting relative to Janice's situation, Scenario 1, follows. The components of outcome-oriented charting are data base (nursing history); problem identification (usual and unusual); desired patient outcomes (clinical and behavioral short-term objectives); deadlines for evaluation and documentation; nursing orders; outcome documentation (progress notes), and standards for discharge or maintenance. The data base is documented in the nursing assessment guide shown in Table 3.1. The problems, expected outcomes, deadlines, nursing orders, and standards for discharge are shown on the care plan in Fig. 3.11.

The outcome-oriented progress notes describe the client's response to care. They show the comparison between the desired and the real client status.

DATE	PROGRESS NOTES
ADMISSION NOTE	
10/12	Home visit — Client is 29-year-old female, 2½ months gestation. Baseline data and identified problems are shown on the nursing history and the care plan.
	A. Johnson, R.N.
INTERIM NOTE	
10/26	Home visit — Janice states that she has decided to have an abortion. She reviewed the pros and cons of this decision and seems willing to adjust to this decision. Expressed feelings of decreased tension by weeping when discussing decision, yet laughing and smiling when thinking about future. Did not discuss long-term goals at this time. Stated that she has been too preoccupied with immediate decision to do any reading or thinking about future relationships with men.
	A. Johnson, R.N.
DISCHARGE SUMMARY	
11/26	Verbalizes that she is working with a counselor regarding some as yet unresolved feelings about having terminated the pregnancy. Expresses that she has had satisfying experiences with the abortion clinic. States that she is deferring long-term life goals to meet immediate need of finding out more about herself. For the same reason she is deferring her prior concerns about future relationships with men. Closed to service.
	A. Johnson, R.N.

Figure 3.12

Care Plan, Scenario Two, Mrs. Ellison

STANDARDS FOR DISCHARGE OR MAINTENANCE: *Verbalizes that she is not anxious about her relationship with husband.*

DATE	PROBLEMS	EXPECTED OUTCOMES	DEADLINES	NURSING ORDERS	COMPLETED
10/2	1. Acute fear due to "unknowns" regarding husband's feelings and uncertainty about outcome of surgery.	1. Verbalizes correct knowledge regarding reasons for surgery. Verbalizes her feeling about relationship with husband.	Before surgery √ daily A.M.	1a. Verify that she has correct knowledge re. surgery prior to surgery. b. Inform physician with client's permission of her concerns this evening. Delegated to M. Berg R.N. c. Spend time actively listening in p.m. before surgery and q̄ a.m. thereafter. M. Berg, R.N.	

Figure 3.13

Updated Care Plan, Scenario Two, Mrs. Ellison

STANDARDS FOR DISCHARGE OR MAINTENANCE: *Verbalizes that she is not anxious about her relationship with husband.*

DATE	PROBLEMS	EXPECTED OUTCOMES	DEADLINES	NURSING ORDERS	SIGNATURE
10/2	Acute fear due to "unknowns" regarding husband's feelings and uncertainty of outcome of surgery.	Verbalizes correct knowledge regarding reasons for surgery.	Before surgery	Verify that she has current knowledge re surgery prior to surgery.	D.C. 10/2 9 P.M. M.B., R.N.
				Inform physician (with client's permission) of her concerns this evening. Delegated to M. Berg, R.N.	D.C. 10/2 9 P.M. M.B., R.N.
10/2	Continued concern regarding husband's possible reaction to effects of surgery.	Verbalizes her feelings about relationship with husband.	√ daily A.M.	Delegated to M. Berg, R.N. Spend time actively listening in p.m. before surgery and q̄ A.M. thereafter.	

Scenario 2

Mrs. Ellison is the person who has been admitted to the gynecological-surgical unit of an acute-care hospital. She is preoperative for a total abdominal hysterectomy. The documentation for her situation is illustrated in source, problem, and outcome-oriented methods.

Table 3.2 (p. 131) shows a nursing assessment guide for Mrs. Ellison. It is limited to the interactive/affiliative system.

Documenting the Planning Process

The care plan developed for Mrs. Ellison is shown in Fig. 3.12. Fig. 3.13 shows the updated care plan reflecting problem resolution and change in focus.

Methods of Charting

Source-Oriented—In illustrating source-oriented charting relative to scenario 2, it is assumed that the care plan is not kept as part of the permanent record. Charting for Mrs. Ellison during three phases of care (admission, interim, and discharge) follows:

DATE	NURSES' NOTES
ADMISSION	
10/2	Admitted client to room 222. Refered to nursing history.
4 P.M.	Discussed concerns. Expresses fear regarding surgery, does not really understand why surgery is indicated. Is afraid of cancer. Feels unable to discuss fears with husband. Suggested that nurse return later this evening to discuss her feelings...client agrees. Also agrees that physician should be notified of her fears. Nursing plans include follow-up on a daily basis regarding husband-wife relationships.
	M. Berg, R.N.
INTERIM	
10/2	Phoned physician and informed of client's fears. Since
9 P.M.	talking with physician, client expresses relief — and is able to discuss reasons for surgery. Husband visited earlier this evening. Appeared supportive, yet client states they didn't really discuss specifics relative to surgery. client agrees to continue to discuss this concern following immediate postoperative period.
	M. Berg, R.N.

| 10/5 9:30 P.M. | Talked with client today regarding her interactions with her husband. She responded by saying he is genuinely concerned about her health — is attentive, but she has not at this time brought up her concerns about her identity as a woman. |
| | N. Austin, R.N. |

DISCHARGE SUMMARY

| 10/8 11 A.M. | Reviewed preexisting concerns about female identity and aftermath of surgery. States she and husband still have not discussed her fears. Suggested referral to counseling services. Client firmly refuses, stating that this is really a normal pattern for them and now that surgery is over she thinks she can handle her feelings. |
| | N. Austin, R.N. |

Problem-Oriented—Mrs. Ellison's situation is documented through the problem-oriented method.

Data Base—Data-base information is illustrated in Table 3.2.

PROBLEM LIST

DATE	ACTIVE PROBLEMS	INACTIVE PROBLEMS
10/2 1 4 PM	Acute fear due to "unknowns" regarding husband's feelings and uncertainty of outcomes of surgery. 10/2 9 AM Resolved	
2		Recurring lumps in breasts. Subjective data. No objective data available.
3	Continued concern regarding husband's possible reaction to effects of surgery. 10/8 11 AM Resolved	

INITIAL PLAN

1. Acute fear due to husband's feelings and uncertainty about outcomes of surgery.

   Diagnostic Plans   Determine correct information;

INITIAL PLAN (cont.)

	verify reasons for surgery. Identify normal husband/wife interaction pattern.
Therapeutic Plans	Active listening. Inform physician with client's knowledge of her concerns.
Patient Education Plans	Teach client specifics regarding reasons for surgery (to be done by physician); postoperative regime and long-term physical and emotional implications.
	M. Berg, R.N.

PROGRESS NOTES

DATE	NO.	PROBLEM	PROGRESS NOTES
INTERIM *10/2* *9 P.M.*	1	Acute fear	S — Expresses relief after talking with physician.
			O — Able to explain reasons for surgery consistent with physician's explanation.
			A — Experiencing less tension relative to surgery; however still unable to discuss with husband.
			P — Discuss concerns on a daily basis after immediate post-op period.
			M. Berg, R.N.
10/5 *9:30 P.M.*	2	Continued concern	S — States she still isn't able to discuss fears with her husband. He is, however, "attentive" and "supportive."
			O — Calm — relaxed countenance.
			A — Seems accepting of existing relationship with husband.
			P — Continue to discuss on a daily basis.

DISCHARGE SUMMARY			
10/8 *11 A.M.*	3	Continued concern	S — States she and husband have not discussed her fears. Refused counseling services, "...thinks she can handle her feelings." O — Tone of voice conveys certainty. Calm mannerisms. A — Conclude that she is not feeling anxious about relationship with husband. P — Discharge from nursing services. M. Berg, R.N.

Outcome-Oriented—The outcome-oriented method of charting for Mrs. Ellison is shown in the subsequent notes. All the components of this method of documentation except these progress notes, appear in Table 3.2 and Figs. 3.12 and 3.13.

DATE	*PROGRESS NOTES*
ADMISSION NOTE *10/2* *4 P.M.*	Admitted to room 222. Baseline data and identified problems appear on the nursing history and the care plan. M. Berg, R.N.
INTERIM NOTE *10/2* *9 P.M.*	Verbalized correct knowledge regarding reasons for surgery. Expressed continued concern regarding relationship with husband. M. Berg, R.N.
10/5 *9:30 P.M*	States that husband is attentive and supportive. Still unable to discuss her concerns with him. M. Berg, R.N.
DISCHARGE SUMMARY *10/8* *11 A.M.*	Expressed that her fears have not yet been discussed with husband, but is now able to handle her feelings; recognizes that this "not-talking" is really a normal pattern for them. No counseling referral indicated. M. Berg, R.N.

AUTOMATION: AID TO DOCUMENTATION

Automation refers to those techniques that simplify or replicate the written word and that aid in the four communication processes of assembling, coding, classifying, and disseminating. Automation may take many forms: it can be as simple as a copying machine, a transcriber, a telecopier, soft carbonized paper; or as complex as a comprehensive computerized information system. Any of these forms may be incorporated into any of the documentation methods discussed in this chapter. Which type of automation to use is dependent upon the goals or purposes of a specific communication process. For example, a patient-care conference may best profit from several xeroxed copies of the care plan, while a pharmacy or admitting department that communicates hundreds of times a day with many departments may profit from some form of computerized documentation system.

The increasing complexity of the developing knowledge base in nursing, as well as requirements and constraints of regulatory bodies, demands that nursing consider the use of sophisticated automation systems. For example, in the educational setting automation can take the form of computerized testing services, auto tutorial learning systems, computerized reference centers, and many other systems. Nurse researchers can take advantage of similar technologies as well as a recently developed concept called tele-conferencing. This computer-assisted mechanism makes it possible for researchers who are geographically separated to maintain constant written communication with their colleagues who share similar work. Within the context of nursing services, "the increasing complexity and quantity of care technologies, the rising average acuity of patients, and the proliferating specialties and specialists...are creating massive demands upon nursing—for coordination, for decision-making and for effective communication."[11] Nurses as well as other professionals waste large amounts of time in finding the information they use and writing it down on forms which are difficult to retrieve later.[12] A computer-assisted information system removes some of the obstacles that stand between an agency's personnel and its possibility for rendering high-quality care. Information systems make available complete and timely information for the decisions that affect clients' well-being. They reduce errors of delay and call attention to the staff's "sometimes overburdened memories or teach them facts that they have not had time to uncover for themselves. A computerized system can enable everyone who comes in contact with it to come closer, perhaps closer than ever before, to achieving one's own potential for providing patient care."[13]

One hospital's computer-assisted nursing information system is described by Cook, Hushower, and Mayers.[11] The nursing service department of El Camino Hospital is a decentralized organization comprised of 16 clinical units, each with a head nurse who reports to the director of nursing services. Each head nurse is responsible for her unit, its patients and staff, on a 24-hour-a-day, seven-day-a-week basis. Each is responsible for achieving specific, measureable management objectives relating to quality care, staff growth and development, and cost-effectiveness. A computerized information system has been implemented at this hospital to aid in achieving these objectives.

The Technicon Medical Information System (TMIS)* was adopted by El Camino Hospital to attack head-on the enormous cost of manual information processing. TMIS is a real-time, comprehensive, integrated medical information system that operates from a large-scale computer located in the vendor's regional center, which is connected to video and printer terminals located throughout the hospital. Doctors, nurses, and other hospital professional and clerical personnel interact directly with the system by use of these terminals to enter, retrieve, and print clinical, financial, and administrative information. TMIS automates, either in whole or in part, a great many of the patient-oriented information-processing tasks that are performed thousands of times daily in a hospital. The system captures patient information from admission through discharge, focusing primarily on the physician's medical order and the subsequent actions required to execute and record the results of this medical order. The system impacts all nursing units and clinical ancillary departments, as well as many administrative and support departments. Care-planning as one form of documentation was computerized and tested at this hospital.

Computerized Care-Planning

All but three or four nursing services in the United States handwrite the plans of care onto cards which are kept in a rand for easy access. Few nursing services are successful in keeping care plans updated, primarily because of the large amounts of detailed, constantly changing information which should be written. This results in nurses giving token attention to the writing of care plans, relying primarily on "word-of-mouth" information transmission. Because in a typical hospital any one client is likely to have 12 to 14 different nurses caring for him over a five-day average hospital stay, the "word-of-mouth" method is fraught with problems of faulty recall and fragmented information. The result is an inadequacy of analysis and planning data available to any nurse as she cares for a client.

The focus of the El Camino Hospital TMIS Care Planning system is that of computerizing outcome-oriented patient care-planning so that the operational difficulties of manipulating large quantities of data can be made efficient enough that care-planning will actually be done by nurses. Outcome-oriented care-planning is also designed so that the computerized data can be used for both concurrent and retrospective audit purposes. The

*Technicon Medical Information Systems Santa Clara, Ca., 95051. A division of Technicon Instruments Corporation.

hospital is seeking to improve the quality of client care and improve the effectiveness with which it is delivered by implementing a computer-assisted outcome-oriented patient care-planning system. The system integrates (a) diagnosis-particular, outcome-oriented standard nursing care plans, (b) outcome-oriented, systematic nursing care-planning processes, and (c) the computerized medical information system in use at this hospital. This integrated system is designed to focus nursing care on client outcomes rather than on nursing tasks, and to compare actual outcomes against standards. This system also produces the necessary data required by a total patient-care audit system.

At the time of the study a pilot unit was fully implemented and two other units were being implemented. The subsequent discussion summarizes the features of the TMIS care-planning system and provides preliminary evaluation data from the pilot-study implementation unit.

Nursing Component

The care-planning process begins when the client arrives at the nursing unit. The first step is an interview. Data from the interview, from other chart documents such as the physician's history and the physical examination, and from the standard care-plans data base resident in the computer is synthesized at the video terminal to produce this patient's care plan, which reflects not only his diagnosis but also his unique problems.

The care plan is formulated in terms of both real problems and potential problems, expected outcomes that reflect the resolution of the problems, deadlines by which this resolution can be reached, and nursing orders representing necessary nursing actions to accomplish this resolution. The problems needing resolution may be either short- or long-range.

The care plan is recorded at the video terminal by selecting the appropriate items from the standard care-plan data base and by typing in any special problem(s) specific to this client. Entering the care plan via the terminal produces a printed version of this individualized plan for use by the nurse caring for the client. This printout includes all care-planning data as well as expected date of discharge estimated by the nurse and the initials of the nurse responsible for the data.

The printed version of the care plan is produced once a day, or on demand, and serves as the nurse's work sheet as she cares for the client. While caring for him, she determines, in conjunction with him, which expected outcomes have been or are being accomplished. She also determines if deadlines are realistic and if the nursing orders are effective.

The information gleaned from caring for the client is documented via TMIS in the nurse's notes and describes the patient's progress toward expected outcomes. At the same time, the nurse can update (via TMIS) the care plan. She "completes" those problems resolved, and if necessary, changes such other data as deadlines or nursing orders to reflect current needs. The next printed care plan reflects these changes. As the client progresses toward recovery, this is reflected in the care plan, as expected outcomes are reached.

The video matrix features of the care plan are as follows:

- Standard care plans (diagnosis-related) are stored in the computer memory bank.
- Standard care plans (SCP's) are easily adapted to each client. Usual or non-standard care plans are easily formulated.
- There are cross-reference indices between standard care plans and problems.
- Lists of real and potential problems are contained within each standard care plan.
- Problems that are common to several standard care plans are standardized and listed separately.
- Abbreviations are incorporated to save time and space.
- Relative deadlines, readily translatable into actual dates for expected outcomes, are provided.
- Coordination between the responsible nurse and the utilization review nurse is facilitated.

The care plan includes the identity of the responsible and alternate nurse; the estimated discharge date; criteria for discharge; real and potential problems; expected outcomes; deadlines; and nursing orders and possible problems which require further data or watchfulness. Fig. 3.14 illustrates a typical matrix sequence. Fig. 3.15 is an example of a common problems list.

The TMIS Care Plan has two sections, a medical care plan (MCP) and a nursing care plan (NCP). These two documents used together constitute a patient care plan and replace the traditional Kardex or Rand file and contain all current information for each patient. They can be printed out at specified times, or on demand, in the required number of copies.

This care plan is used as the individual nurse's worksheet in order to implement medical and nursing care; assign staff; take and give reports; annotate for charting; and perform evaluations and nursing audits. The care plan is applicable to any mode of nursing-care delivery, i.e., primary, team, case method. The patient care plan extends to or interfaces with charting; evaluation/nursing audit; nurse staffing; utilization review; and diagnosis coding.

The special features of the care plan are several:

- They are printed on request, as needed, due to changes in client status.
- The plan encompasses all current problems.
- Plans are updated as problems, expected outcomes, deadlines, or nursing orders are added, deleted, or revised.

120

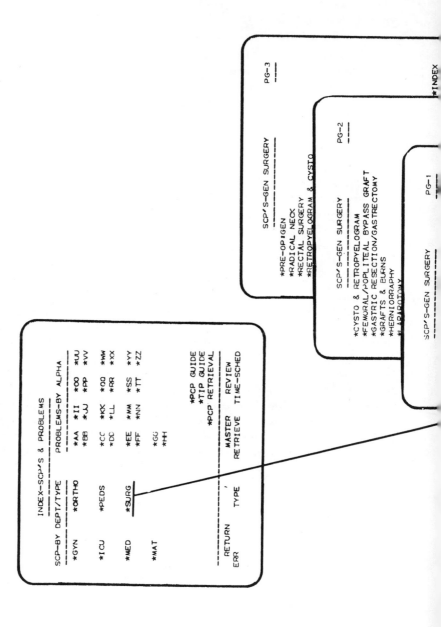

Figure 3.14
Typical Matrix Sequence

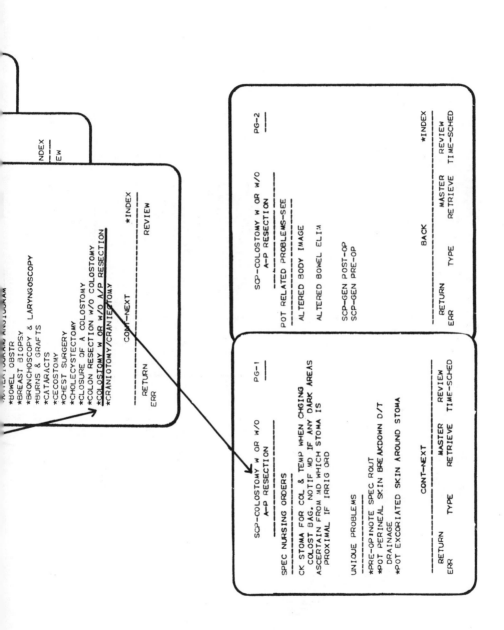

Figure 3.15
Common Problems List

```
COMMON PROBLEMS:A                    PG-1
----------------                     ----
*ADL ROUT
(AIRWAY:SEE POT LOSS OF PATENT AIRWAY)
(ACTIV:SEE INTOLERANCE OF ACTIV)
*ADVERSE PHYSIO CHG D/T DELIV
*ADVERSE REACTION TO ANES
*ALTERED BLADDER CONTROL
..(D/T SPINAL CORD INJURY)
*ALTERED BODY IMAGE
*ALTERED BOWEL ELIM
(ALTERED CONSCIOUSNESS:SEE CONFUSION,
..ALTERED CONSCIOUSNESS)
*ALT INSULIN NEEDS W METABOLIC DEM OF PG
*ALTERED SENSATION
*ALTERED URIN ELIM
(AMBULATION:SEE IMPAIRED MOBILITY:POT
..UNSAFE AMB)
*ANGER/HOSTILITY
            CONT-NEXT         *INDEX
------------           -------------
RETURN                 REVIEW
ERR
```

Figure 3.16
Example of Computerized Care Plan

```
ALTERED BODY IMAGE            PG-1
                              ----
POT REAL D/T---

EXPECTED OUTCOMES,DOC'S,EDL'S
----------------------------
V & DEMO INTEREST IN APPEARANCE
  & PROGRESS   (DOC)____ (EDL)____
V CONCERN RE:CLOSE PERSONAL
  RELATINSHIPS  (DCC)____ (EDL)____
V PLANS FOR PROSTH (DOC)____ (EDL)____

OTHER EO---      (DOC)____ (EDL)____

NURSING ORDERS
-------------
DELEGATE 1-RN TO SPEND TIME INTERACTING
  W PT RE:FEELINGS
DISCUSS APPROP RESOURCE PEOPLE W MD & PT
ENC PT TO ATTAIN POSITIVE BODY IMAGE
  (HAIR GROOMING,COSMETICS,GOWN,SHAVING)
ALLOW SIGNIF OTHER TO EXPRESS CONCERNS,&
  HELP PROBLEM-SOLVE
MINIMIZE OFFENSIVE ODORS
CHG DSG IMMED WHEN SOILED

OTHER NO---

                                      **
-----------      BACK          *INDEX
RETURN                         REVIEW
ERR
```

- The plans focus on the outcomes of care (expected outcomes) as well as the required nursing interventions (orders).
- A summary care plan is printed after the client is discharged. The summary plan lists all problems and their components during the hospital stay; is used for post-discharge evaluation (nursing audit) purposes; may be filed with the chart for reference in the event of readmission, or for research and education purposes.

Fig. 3.16 is an example of a computerized care plan.

Medical Component

The medical care plan includes medical orders grouped into the following categories: vital signs; diet and fluid balance; unit tests/examinations; and miscellaneous orders. Also included are "test prep" categories. The features of the medical care plan are:

- All current medical orders and test preps are on the plan. Orders are complete, legible, unambiguous.
- Medical orders that appear on medical care plans are entered at the video matrix terminal (VMT) by either physician or nurse.
- Expired drug orders and floor-stocked drugs are "flagged."
- They are routinely printed in advance of each shift.
- The medical plan is reviewed and updated each shift to maintain its currency.

Evaluation

The computerized care-planning system just described was pilot-tested on a 40-bed orthopedic unit. The objectives of the pilot test were:

1. Improved quality of planning, charting, and evaluation of client care (outcome-oriented); comprehensiveness; currency; and relevancy.
2. Increased ease of access to a memory bank library of standard care plans, problem lists, and care protocols.
3. Increased quality in the charting of client progress (outcome-related; comprehensive yet concise; and deadline-related).
4. Increased integration of physician- and nurse-initiated plans.
5. No increase in nursing labor costs attributable to the care-planning system.

The pilot unit evaluation took the form of a pre (T_1) and post (T_2) test design. A structured questionnaire to members of the pilot unit staff provided much of the evaluative data. A comparison of nursing hours per patient day provided labor-cost information; and bedside and chart audits provided additional objective data.

When this system of care-planning was implemented on the pilot unit a number of results became evident. On the positive side, there was a distinct increase in the amount of care-planning, averaging 82 percent of patients with a care plan. This led to greater consistency in patient care. These care plans were current at least 85 percent of the time. With this increase in planning of care, charting began to reflect patient outcomes, and discharge planning was initiated earlier in the patient's stay. An indirect result was that the nurses were able to rate the patient's need for nursing care (required labor hours) on a more consistent basis.

One result of the pilot study was some system redesign. Prior to redesign, it was easier to select all data from a standard care plan rather than to select only what was appropriate to the individual client. This led nurses often to choose the easier, less accurate method. After minor system redesign, the care plans more nearly reflect the clients' problems.

Initial system design also encouraged entering and printing a large volume of data. This has been corrected through modifying system designs and by some retraining of personnel.

Labor-analysis findings revealed that there were no increases in nursing labor costs that could be attributable to the TMIS computerized care planning system.

Table 3.1

Interactive/Affiliative System:
Assessment Guide, Janice, Scenario 1

- Interpersonal Theories

STANDARD 1. Presence of feelings of security in most important interpersonal relationships.

INFERENCES
Met
Not Met √

VALIDATION
Agreed √
Disagreed

NURSING DIAGNOSIS (DEDUCTION)
Constant insecurity due to conflict between self-expectations and achievements and whether or not to terminate pregnancy.

Questions, Observations, Examinations	Client Responses
1. How do you feel about what is happening to you? Put down Not recognized or valued	1. Confused, upset, not ready, depressed over unplanned pregnancy.
2. Do you feel you have control over what is happening to you?	2. Feels like a victim. A lot of life seems to happen by accident.
3. Has something like this ever happend to you before; what do you remember about it?	3. Not exactly. Depressed.
4. Who, if anyone, can help you (be supportive to you) at this time?	4. Mother and sister.
5. Who are the important people in your life? Family Significant Others Work Group Social Group	5. Sister. Associated with a work group.

Table 3.1 *(cont.)*
Interactive/Affiliative System:
Assessment Guide, Janice, Scenario 1

Questions, Observations, Examinations	Client Responses
6. Do relationships with these people make you feel *comfortable, uncomfortable?* Now Past Potential in Future	6. *Comfortable.*

7. What interactions, if any, tend to upset you?
• Observations
  Body Language
  Posture
  Muscle tension
  Random/compulsive movements
  Tone of voice
	7. *With ex-boyfriend*
	
	Occasional change from relaxed to upright. Frequent movement of hands/feet; clasping, unclasping hands. Long heavy sighs. Strong, clear, emphatic answers.

• Communication Theories	
INFERENCES	NURSING DIAGNOSIS (DEDUCTION)
STANDARD 2. Ability to change behavior of self or others in an attempt to reduce uncertainty. Met √ Not Met	VALIDATION Agreed √ Disagreed
STANDARD 3. Ability to communicate in interpersonal and group relationships. Met √ Not Met	Agreed √ Disagreed

Questions, Observations, Examinations	Client Responses
8. How do you usually find out what others expect of you?	8. Asks — double checks. Sometimes guesses.
9. How easy or difficult is it for you to follow through?	9. Easy, challenging.
10. In your past, how have you been able to respond to your own or others' expectations?	10. "My family thinks I'm great." Not too secure about social relationships.
11. Do you usually feel in control of the situation or a victim of the circumstances?	11. Usually feels in control. Not right now — ambivalent about future of pregnancy — should she keep the baby?
12. How have you generally responded to pressures for change in your life style?	12. Usually does what has to be done — now feels anxious.
13. What type of work do you do?	13. Personnel — section manager.
14. How do you spend your leisure time?	14. Frittering away — seems to enjoy self. Reading — Traveling.
15. How do you feel about your achievements in life?	15. Rather incredible. Halfway toward college degree while working — others view as successful — agrees.
16. What important things do you feel you have accomplished?	16. See above.
• Observations Transmitting ideas clearly Receiving or understanding Validating or checking out	Clear emphatic answers. Yes. Yes.

Table 3.1 (cont.)
Interactive/Affiliative System:
Assessment Guide, Janice, Scenario 1

Questions, Observations, Examinations		Client Responses	
			NURSING DIAGNOSIS (DEDUCTION)
• Group/Role Theories			
STANDARD 4. Membership in one or more social groups.	INFERENCES Met ✓ Not Met	VALIDATION Agreed ✓ Disagreed	
STANDARD 5. Membership in a kin network.	Met ✓ Not Met	Agreed ✓ Disagreed	
STANDARD 6. Perceived sense of comfort with values and norms of reference groups.	Met Not Met ✓ *Potential conflict with mother, fear of rejection.*	Agreed Disagreed ✓ *Client says mother will be supportive.*	*Inference not substantiated by client.*
STANDARD 7. Ability to rank loyalties among reference groups.	Met ✓ Not Met	Agreed ✓ Disagreed	
STANDARD 8. Satisfaction with role identity.	Met Not Met ✓	Agreed ✓ Disagreed	*Sudden role ambivalency due to unplanned pregnancy.*

Questions, Observations, Examinations	Client Responses
17. Is there someone/s on whom you rely?	17. *Primarily sister.*
18. How easy is it to keep in touch with those who are important to you?	18. *Very easy — lives nearby. Mother by phone.*

19. What groups are you affiliated with?

19. *None right now — just work.*

20. Which do you feel most comfortable with?

20. *Comfortable with work group.*

21. How consistent are your opinions and feelings with those in the group?

21. *Agrees most of the time. Unsure of mother's reaction to pregnancy. May be conflict of values.*

22. Which groups are the most important to you?

22. *Work group*

23. How able are you to meet their expectations?

23. *Okay — fine.*

24. How many roles do you assume right now in your life?

24. *Career girl, boss, student, sister, and feels like a mother already — some ambivalence noted.*

25. Which role is most important?

25. *None of those — something else. Desired role as a "person."*

26. Are you satisfied with this role?

26. *Not really — again expresses conflict over decision as to future of pregnancy — baby.*

• Observations
  Body Language
  Posture
  Muscle tension
  Random/compulsive movements
  Tone of voice

Nervous laughter.

• Intimacy Theories:

STANDARD 9. Closeness with another throughout life.

INFERENCES	VALIDATION
Met	Agreed √
Not Met √	Disagreed

NURSING
DIAGNOSIS
(DEDUCTION)

Uncertainty due to change in future role and establishing a relationship with another man.

Table 3.1 *(cont.)*
Interactive/Affiliative System:
Assessment Guide, Janice, Scenario 1

Questions, Observations, Examinations			Client Responses
27. What about close personal relationship in your life?			27. Some feelings toward former boyfriend — no one else at present. Decided to dismiss him from life. Feels loss of man in life. Relies on sister now.
• Culture Theories:			NURSING DIAGNOSIS (DEDUCTION)
STANDARD 10. A state of being consistent with the values, norms, and goals of most important reference groups.	INFERENCES Met √ Not Met	VALIDATION Agreed √ Disagreed	See Standard 6.
Questions, Observations, Examinations			Client Responses
Refer back to previous questions related to group/role.			

Table 3.2

Interactive/Affiliative System:
Assessment Guide, Mrs. Ellison

• Interpersonal Theories:

STANDARD 1. Presence of feelings of security in most important interpersonal relationships.

INFERENCES	VALIDATION	NURSING DIAGNOSIS (DEDUCTION)
Met √ Not Met	Agreed Disagreed √	Acute fear due to "unknowns" regarding husband's feelings and uncertainty about outcomes of surgery.

Questions, Observations, Examinations	Client Responses
1. How do you feel about what is happening to you? Put down Not recognized or valued	1. Scared, really scared. Frightened of cancer. Afraid surgery might interfere with marriage.
2. Do you feel you have control over what is happening to you?	2. No — everything is going too fast. Feeling a little sorry for self. Not sure of necessity for surgery.
3. Has something like this ever happened to you before; what do you remember about it?	3. Prior concern about lump in breast. Recurrent feelings of fear.
4. Who, if anyone, can help you (be supportive to you) at this time?	4. Husband, maybe? Afraid to discuss with him. Mother and sister — not in immediate area.

Table 3.2 *(cont.)*

Interactive/Affiliative System:
Assessment Guide, Mrs. Ellison

Questions, Observations, Examinations	Client Responses
5. Who are the important people in your life? 　　Family 　　Significant Others 　　Work Group 　　Social Group	5. *Family — definitely.* *Work friends* *Social friends*
6. Do relationships with these people make you feel comfortable/uncomfortable? 　　Now 　　Past 　　Potential in future	6. *Good*
7. What interactions, if any, tend to upset you? ● Observations 　　Body Language 　　Posture 　　Muscle tension 　　Random/compulsive 　　movements 　　Tone of voice	7. *Unable to discuss surgery with husband.* *Unchanged — looks straight ahead rather than at interviewer. Voice calm — spoke rapidly when mentioning concern over husband.*

• Communication Theories:

	INFERENCES	VALIDATION	NURSING DIAGNOSIS (DEDUCTION)
STANDARD 2. Ability to change behavior of self or others in an attempt to reduce uncertainty.	Met √ Not Met	Agreed √ Disagreed	
STANDARD 3. Ability to communicate in interpersonal and group relationships.	Met √ Not Met	Agreed √ Disagreed	

Questions, Observations, Examinations	Client Responses
8. How do you usually find out what others expect of you?	8. People tend to turn to her for help.
9. How easy or difficult is it for you to follow through?	9. Able to follow through.
10. In your past, how have you been able to respond to your own or others' expectations?	10. Competent — able, but feels stressed due to many demands.
11. Do you usually feel in control of the situation or a victim of the circumstances?	11. Usually in control except for right now. Expresses concern for time for self in the future.
12. How have you generally responded to pressures for change in your life style?	12. Initiates own changes rather than responding to pressures for change.
13. What type of work do you do?	13. Librarian
14. How do you spend your lesiure time?	14. Son, school and social activity, dancing, reading, bicycling, tennis.
15. How do you feel about your achievements in life?	15. Very satisfied.

Table 3.2 *(cont.)*
Interactive/Affiliative System:
Assessment Guide, Mrs. Ellison

Questions, Observations, Examinations			Client Responses
16. What important things do you feel you have accomplished?			16. *Prestige in professional setting — family role.*
• Observations			
Transmitting ideas clearly.			*Articulate.*
Receiving or understanding.			*Yes.*
Validating or checking out.			*Yes.*
• Group/Role Theories:	INFERENCES		VALIDATION
STANDARD 4. Membership in one or more social groups.	Met √	Not Met	Agreed √ / Disagreed
STANDARD 5. Membership in a kin network.	Met √	Not Met	Agreed √ / Disagreed
STANDARD 6. Perceived sense of comfort with values and norms of reference groups.	Met √	Not Met	Agreed √ / Disagreed
STANDARD 7. Ability to rank loyalties among reference groups.	Met √	Not Met	Agreed √ / Disagreed

NURSING
DIAGNOSIS
(DEDUCTION)

STANDARD 8. Satisfaction with role identity.

Met	Not Met √	Agreed	Disagreed √	Inference not substantiated
	Suppressing own emotional need due to family demands.		Client prefers to maintain existing pattern.	by client.

Questions, Observations, Examinations	Client Responses
17. Is there someone/s on whom you rely?	17. Husband.
18. How easy is it to keep in touch with those who are important to you?	18. Husband — at home. Family within reach by long-distance phone.
19. What groups are you affiliated with?	19. Family. Work & Profession. Boy Scouts. Social.
20. Which do you feel most comfortable with?	20. Family
21. How consistent are your opinions and feelings with those in the group?	21. Okay with consistency but not enough energy to continually meet all of these demands — wants to continue, however.
22. Which groups are the most important to you?	22. Family — then work.
23. How able are you to meet their expectations?	23. Able, but not enough energy to continually meet all demands — seems angry as friends don't reciprocate to support but will continue to keep this pattern.
24. How many roles do you assume right now in your life?	24. Wife, mother, librarian, friend.
25. Which role is most important?	25. Wife and mother.
26. Are you satisfied with this role?	26. Yes — and no. Angry because she "does not have enough time to be me."

Table 3.2 *(cont.)*
Interactive/Affiliative System:
Assessment Guide, Mrs. Ellison

Questions, Observations, Examinations		Client Responses	
• Observations			
Body Language			
Posture			
Muscle tension			
Random/compulsive movements			
Tone of voice		*Speaking rapidly without pause.*	
• Intimacy Theories:			NURSING DIAGNOSIS (DEDUCTION)
STANDARD 9. Closeness with another throughout life.	INFERENCES Met √ Not Met	VALIDATION Agreed Disagreed √ *Unable to openly talk with husband — afraid.*	See Standard #1.

Questions, Observations, Examinations		Client Responses	
27. What about close personal relationships in your life?		27. Husband becoming a very special person. "Can't imagine life without him."	
• Culture Theories:			NURSING DIAGNOSIS (DEDUCTION)
STANDARD 10. A state of being consistent with the values, norms, and goals of most important reference groups.	INFERENCES Met √ Not Met	VALIDATION Agreed √ Disagreed	

Questions, Observations, Inspections		Client Responses	

Refer back to previous questions related to group/role.

REFERENCES

1. *Webster's Seventh New Collegiate Dictionary.* Springfield, Mass, G and C Merriam Co, Publishers, 1970, p 246.
2. Robbins S: *The Administrative Process: Integrating Theory and Practice.* Englewood Cliffs, NJ, Prentice-Hall, Inc, 1976, p 396.
3. Murray M: *Fundamentals of Nursing.* Englewood Cliffs, NJ, Prentice-Hall, Inc, 1976, p 136.
4. Weed L: Medical Records, *Medical Education and Patient Care: The Problem Oriented Record as a Basic Tool.* Cleveland, Press of Case Western Reserve University, 1971, p 62.
5. Yarnall S, Atwood J: Problem oriented practice for nurses and physicians: general concepts. *Nurs Clin North Am* 9:2:220, June 1974.
6. Mayers M, Norby R, Watson A: *Quality Assurance for Patient Care. Nursing Perspectives.* New York, Appleton-Century-Crofts, 1977, pp 129, 131, 150.
7. Kemp J: *Instructional Design, A Plan for Unit and Course Development.* Belmont, Calif, Fearon Publishers, 1971, p 23-24.
8. Mager R: *Preparing Instructional Objectives.* Palo Alto, Calif, Fearon Publishers, 1962, p 12.
9. Watson A, Mayers M: *Care Planning: Chronic Problem/Stat Solution.* Stockton, Calif, K/P Co Medical Systems, 1976, p 62.
10. Berni R, Readey H: *Problem Oriented Medical Record Implementation, Allied Health Peer Review.* St Louis, CV Mosby Co, 1974, pp 59.
11. Cook M, Hushower, G, Mayers M: Computerized nursing and TMIS. *Advances in Automated Analysis,* Vol 1, Tarrytown, NY, Mediad Inc, 1976, p 399.
12. Keating F: We mean to have a part of it. *The May Alumnus* 2:1:58, January 1966.
13. Hodge M: *Medical Information Systems, A Resource for Hospitals.* Germantown, Md, Aspen Systems Corp, 1972, p 50.

BIBLIOGRAPHY

Ainsworth T: American Hospital Association's Quality Control Program, American Medical Association Peer Review Program, and the Social Security Ammendments for PSRO's in *Quality Assurance for Nursing Care, Proceedings of an Institute,* Kansas City, Mo, American Nurses' Assoc, October 1973, p 60-76.

Barker M: The era of the computer and its impact on nursing. *Superv Nurse* 2:26-36, 1971.

Birckhead L: Nursing and the technetronic age. *J Nurs Adm* 7:2:16-19, February 1978.

Bleich H: The computer as a consultant. *N Eng J Med* 284:144-147, 1971.

Bristow O, Stickney C, Thompson S: *Discharge Planning for Continuity of Care.* New York, National League for Nursing, 1976.

Cohn S, Fulcher A, Gustafson N: Reliability study of a nursing flow sheet. *J Nurs Adm* 5:30-33, November-December 1975.

Collingwood M: The nursing care plan as a basis for an information system based on individualized patient care. *Nurs Times* 71:12:21-22, 1975.

Cook M: Changing to an automated information system. *Am J Nurs* 75:1:46-51, January 1975.

David J et al: *Guidelines for Discharge Planning.* Rev ed, Thorofare, NJ, Charles B Slack Inc, Publisher, 1973.

Hannah K: The computer and nursing practice. *Nurs Outlook* 24:9:555-558, September 1976.

Hurst J, Walker H (eds): *The Problem-Oriented System.* New York, Medicom Press, 1972.

Little D, Carnevali D: *Nursing Care Planning.* 2nd ed. Philadelphia, JB Lippincott Co, 1976.

Mayers M: *A Systematic Approach to the Nursing Care Plan.* 2nd ed, New York, Appleton-Century-Crofts, 1978.

Quality Control in the Hospital Discharge Survey. Rockville, Md, United States Department of Health, Education, and Welfare, December 1975.

Rodnick J: The use of automated ambulatory medical records. *J Fam Pract* 5:2:253-264, August 1977.

Walter J, Pardee G, Molbo D (eds): *Dynamics of Problem-Oriented Approaches: Patient Care and Documentation.* Philadelphia, JB Lippincott Co, 1976.

Watson A, Mayers M: *Care Planning: Chronic Problem/Stat Solution.* Stockton, Calif, K/P Co Medical Systems, 1976.

Zielstorff R: Nurses can affect computer systems. *J Nurs Adm* 7:3:49-50, March 1978.

4

Practical Applications

In this chapter the principles of assessment and documentation are explained and applied to a variety of nurse-client situations. The entire process of using frameworks, theories, criteria, assessment guides, and various documentation methods is presented.

Let us assume that the nurse is a practitioner in an agency where a conceptual framework similar to the one developed in this book is being used. Let us also assume that complete assessment guides, questions, inspections, and observations have been developed and are easily available in a manual. Of the hundreds of questions, inspections, and observations which ones will she focus on to use?

FOCUS THROUGH ALGORITHMS

An algorithm is a series of steps followed in a logical order that sorts information, progressing from general to specific. Algorithms are sometimes referred to as "branching logic." This is a type of logic that provides a few major-decision choices first; then, depending upon that major choice, follows a logical pathway with increasingly more specific decision junctions down the way.

Algorithms serve as road maps through a maze of data by providing signs or rules for making decisions which efficiently lead to the right decision goal—the client's concerns.

Fig. 4.1 is a flow diagram showing the logic of an assessment algorithm. The nurse finds herself in a situation with a client. She determines, through observing and asking general grand-tour questions, a general focus, a theme for further attention. What she observes and what the client tells her leads her to speculate about which of the systems of man and environment is the most likely area of concern. She follows her path of speculation by asking second-level grand-tour questions* related to that system. If the client's

---

Second-level grand-tour questions were developed by reviewing the theories in each system of man. This review led to the identification of themes that arose from one or a combination of theories. Themes guided the authors to formulate more specific (second-level) grand-tour questions that would be likely to elicit responses relating to the themes. For example, the theories used to interpret the cognitive/intellectual system suggest the following themes: self-awareness; selectivity; control of environment; mastery; competence; a wide range of cognitive skills; skills necessary to achieve one's own end; and control of impulses. These second-level grand-tour questions related to the themes of the congitive/intellectual system, as well as to all the other systems of man and his environment, are found in Table 4.1.

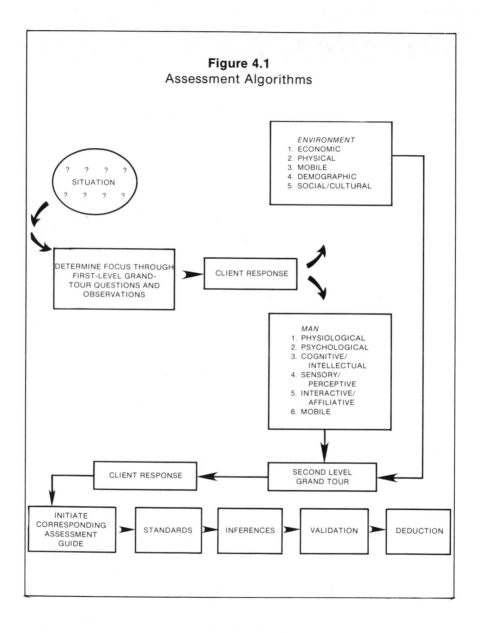

Figure 4.1
Assessment Algorithms

responses confirm her speculation, proceed to the specific assessment guide for that system. As she obtains specific information, she proceeds through the "standards, inferences, validation, and deduction" process. If, at any point in the process, her speculations or inferences are not confirmed, she goes back to the previous decision point and starts down another path.

One of the crucial decision points occurs at the second level when she must speculate as to which system of man is the most likely focus of concern. Validation is absolutely necessary to avoid pursuing the wrong path (choosing the wrong system of man). Some second-level grand-tour questions have been formulated that are designed to increase the nurse's chances of making the right decision at this point. Table 4.1 (p. 176) presents second-level grand-tour questions for the six systems of man, and questions relative to how man is adapting to the five systems of the environment. Table 4.2 (p. 180) illustrates second-level grand-tour questions designed to facilitate and environmental assessment.

In most typical cases in nursing, the primary focus of attention is likely to be man as the client. However, in other cases the environment may, in effect, be the primary focus. In all cases, both man and his environment as open, interactive systems are likely to be the "client."

MAN and environment = Man's health

ENVIRONMENT and man = Environment's health

Situational Applications

A given situation often governs which type of opening grand-tour question will be useful. An acute physical emergency certainly dictates immediate physical assessment and probably precludes questions, observations, and inspections relative to other systems of man. In situations where the focus is not obvious, general grand-tour questions provide both an entree into the situation and a beginning set of data. General grand-tour questions can take the form of statements that respond to non-verbal elements of a situation. Such a grand-tour statement might be: "You seem very busy today." This statement invites a response by the client.

It is important to allow the client to bring up the topics most important to him. The nurse's responses are designed to help the client describe his values and ideas, how he copes or functions, how he thinks about life, and who in the situation is most important to him as his referent group.

Man as the Client

The following situations illustrate the use of a variety of grand-tour questions which lead the nurse to conclude which system of man, and which of the theories within that system, reflect the client's focus of concern.

Situation A—Mrs. Graves is 36 years old and walks into the emergency room unaccompanied. She appears generally ill. The triage nurse asks the following questions.

General
  grand tour   What caused you to come here today?

                    Mrs. Graves: "My sister told me that she thinks I am physically sick and that I should see a doctor."

Physiological
  grand tour   Nurse: "Can you describe how you feel?"

                    Mrs. Graves: "I think I have the flu — I have been home in bed for the last week. I feel sick to my stomach. I can't eat... I have a continuous pain in my stomach and I have chills and fever."

Analysis:	The nurse has received enough information to speculate that Mrs. Graves should be assessed through a physiological systems review. The theories she has in mind are open systems (physiological)[1] and Selye's theory of stress.[2]

Fig. 4.2 is an algorithm that summarizes the decision process used by the nurse to establish the focus of Mrs. Graves' physiological concerns.

Situation B—Mrs. Lancer is 39 years old, with a medical diagnosis of cancer of the liver. She has been told of the diagnosis and the fact that she will start radiation therapy within the week. Currently, she is on intravenous therapy, able to participate in her own care, and is ambulatory. Steve Graham, R.N. will be responsible for her care while she is hospitalized. Having introduced himself, he is proceeding with the nursing assessment. On entering the room he observes Mrs. Lancer lying in bed, hands trembling as she fidgets with the bed covers; the television set is on, several magazines are lying on the bed. Her facial expression is drawn and her brows are knit.

General
  grand tour   Observation of non-verbal situation

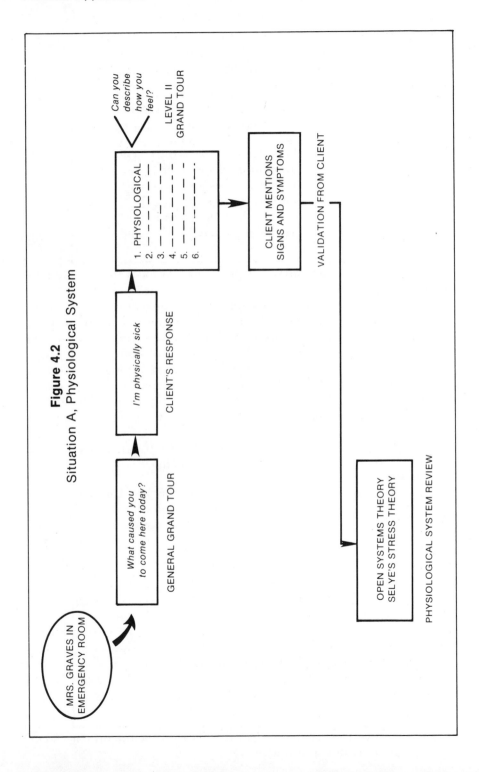

Figure 4.2
Situation A, Physiological System

Psychological grand tour	Nurse:	"There seems to be something bothering you."
	Mrs. Lancer:	Starting to cry: "Everything is wrong. I feel awful. How can I ever get through this? It just isn't fair."

Analysis:	The nurse has now received enough information to speculate about which questions are necessary to complete the assessment. The questions are derived from the theories of anxiety,[3] stress,[2] and grief.[4]

The logic used to determine the psychological focus in Mrs. Lancer's situation is shown in Fig. 4.3.

Situation C—Miss Elder is a 71-year-old lady, a retired nurse, who has been hospitalized for several days. She has been on anticoagulant therapy, receiving heparin intravenously. She had coumadin added to her anticoagulant regime 24 hours earlier. At change of shift, it was reported that Miss Elder had seemed agitated and kept asking when her doctor would be in again. She has been calling the nurses frequently and has been lashing out at them. The nurse decides to assess the meaning of Miss Elder's behavior. She begins the assessment by using a grand-tour question.

General grand tour	Nurse:	"Miss Elder, what difficulties are you experiencing?"
Cognitive/ Intellectual System	Miss Elder:	"I'm worried because I have never seen heparin and coumadin given to a patient at the same time. I thought that I was all through with heparin, but the nurse gave it to me again. I don't know what is wrong. You are not telling me everything."

Analysis:	The nurse has enough information to recognize that the cognitive/ intellectual system of man is involved. She is considering assessment questions related to Lewin's theory of learning[5] and Festinger's theory of cognitive dissonance.[6]

The cognitive/intellectual System is assessed to be the primary focus. The algorithm is shown in Fig. 4.4.

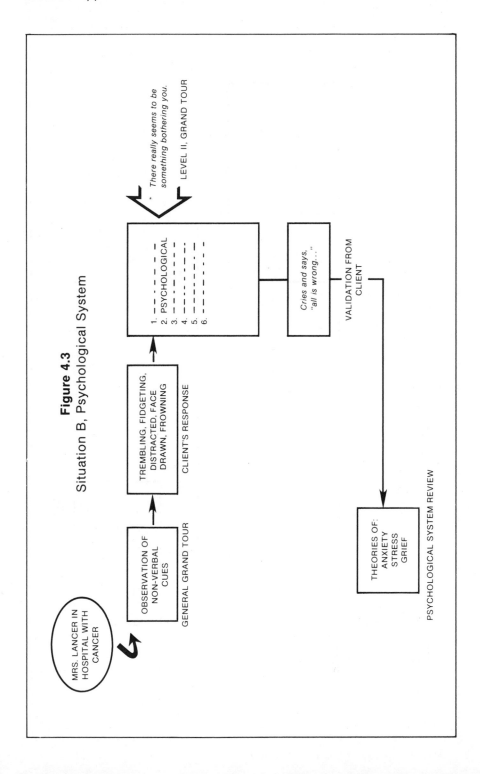

Figure 4.3
Situation B, Psychological System

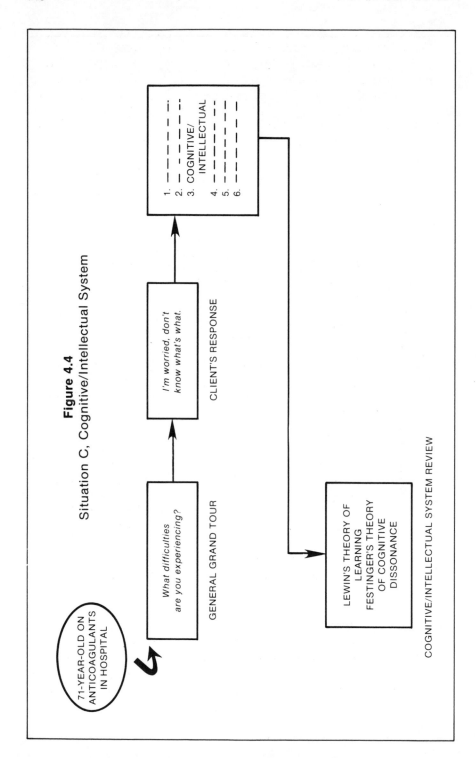

Figure 4.4
Situation C, Cognitive/Intellectual System

Situation D—Mr. Loner is a 44-year-old man who lives by himself in the country. The public-health inspector has visited the premises as a result of complaints from neighbors. They asserted that Mr. Loner kept large numbers of dogs and goats who appeared to be starving. The inspector, while making his investigation, noticed many large draining lesions on the man's face, arms, and hands. For that reason he made a referral to the public-health nurse.

General
grand tour Nurse: "Are you having some problems?"

Mr. Loner: "No — I was just fine until that investigator showed up. I was just minding my own business and now they tell me I have to get rid of my animals, the only real friends I have."

Sensory/
Perceptive Nurse: "Do you understand what is happen-
grand tour ing to you?"

Mr. Loner: "Yes — I understand. They think they're going to take my animals away. Well, that's what they think. I'm going to fight them all the way."

Analysis: The nurse has enough information to recognize that Mr. Loner is experiencing conflict between his perceptions and values and those of society. This leads her to assess further relative to Day's theory of sensory perception.[7]

Fig. 4.5 depicts the process used in arriving at Mr. Loner's concerns.
Situation E—Mrs. Partee is a young woman, age 26, who has delivered her first baby, a healthy girl. She is one day post-partum and is sharing a room with another lady who is also one day post-partum. Mrs. Partee comes from a close-knit upper-middle-class family. She and her husband do not have any family in the immediate area. Mrs. Partee occupies the bed by the door. She tends to keep the curtain drawn between the two beds and faces the door, keeping her back to her roommate. The nurse observes the situation and decides to assess it further.

General
grand tour Observation of non-verbal situation

148

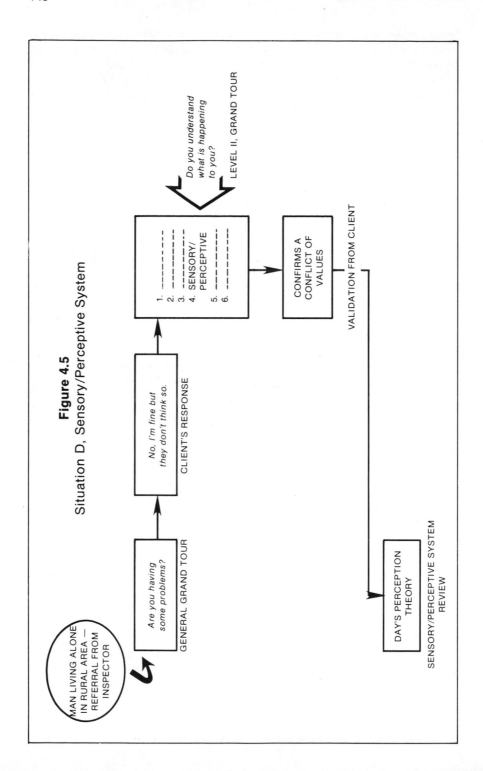

Figure 4.5
Situation D, Sensory/Perceptive System

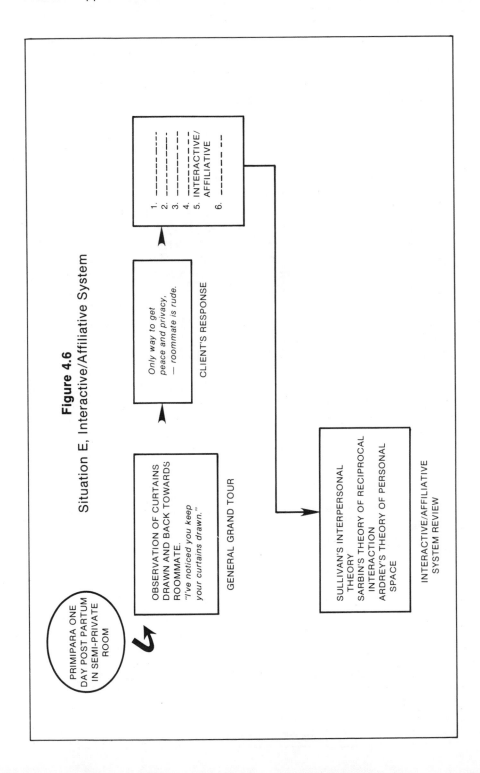

Figure 4.6

Situation E, Interactive/Affiliative System

| | Nurse: | "You know Mrs. Partee, I've noticed that you keep your curtain drawn." |
| Interactive/ Affiliative System | Mrs. Partee: | "It's the only way to get any peace around here. I'm not accustomed to sharing a room with a stranger. It seems too close — and I don't have any privacy. And what's more, she was rude to me last night." |

| Analysis: | The nurse has received enough information cues to query further relative to interactive/affiliative theories: Sullivan's interpersonal theory,[8] Sarbin's theory of reciprocal interaction,[9] and Ardrey's theory of personal space.[10] |

The thought process used to determine the interactive/affiliative focus in Mrs. Partee's situation is shown in Fig. 4.6.

Situation F—Mr. Poore lives on the eighth floor of a low-income housing project. He is 82 years old and shares an apartment with his 78-year-old wife. Both are feeble, but they can usually maintain activities of daily living. The community health nurse visits them monthly to supervise their health care regime. It has been two weeks since her last visit and she receives a phone call.

General grand tour	Nurse:	"I'm surprised to hear from you. Are you having problems?"
	Mr. Poore:	"Yes, the elevators aren't working."
Mobility grand tour	Nurse:	"Are you and your wife able to get about as you need under the circumstances?"
	Mr. Poore:	"No, that's why I'm calling. We're out of groceries. I haven't been able to get my pills for two days. We can't even get out to the park. And I think my wife is getting sick."

| Analysis: | The nurse has received some basic informational cues that leads her to continue an assessment based on Barsch's theory of mobility.[11] |

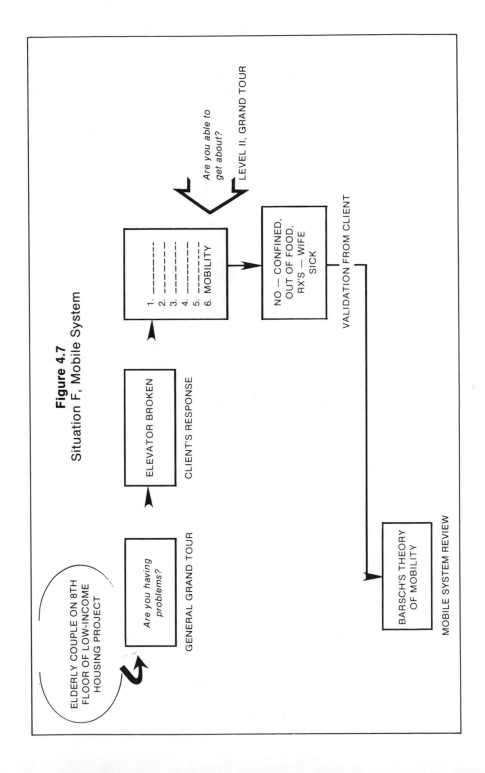

Figure 4.7
Situation F, Mobile System

The mobile system is assessed to be the primary focus. The algorithm is shown in Fig. 4.7.

In each of these situations, the nurse will probably proceed by completing her assessment, using specific questions, observations, and inspections such as those outlined in the assessment guides for the specific concepts or systems of man and the environment. (Examples of such assessment guides are found in the Appendix.)

Environment as the Client

Grand-tour questions or observations can also be used to begin an environmental assessment. This kind of approach focuses on the environment as a client. For example, a community health nurse can assess her region or district for:

Economic Status:	Existing standard of living, supply-and-demand characteristics.
Physical Status:	Quality of air and water, presence of hazards such as noise, chemicals, microbes, and safety.
Mobility Status:	Presence or absence of transit systems.
Demographic Status:	Population density, density characteristics.
Social/Culture Status:	Presence or absence of stimuli and security, prevailing habits and trends for dealing with life.

Environmental assessment is a universal concept in that it is equally important for the nurse who practices within the walls of an agency as in the community. For example, an economic assessment of a patient-care unit requires one to look at its resources—financial, material, and human—and its processes of technology and specialization. Physical assessment might include the quality of air and water (such as the ever-broken ice machine) and noise levels (patient-to-patient, high density of staff contributing to noise). Similar assessments can be made for the remaining systems of the environment. Situations A and B show two of the other systems.

Situation A—Meg Butler, P.H.N. has a new district. It is downtown in a large city and covers a 14-square-block area.

General grand tour	Nurse's observations: Drives through the district and makes some general observations. There are wall-to-wall buildings six to 12 stories high, 30 to 60 years old; litter is scattered about.

	During the day a few older people and a few unkempt young people are walking about, most of them alone. Automobile traffic is heavy. A few small "mama-and-papa" grocery stores appear. In the early evening young girls are grouped on street corners. A few long, low limousines are cruising about.
Demographic grand tour	

> Analysis: Meg, the P.H.N. has made observations which lead her to speculate that the demographic system of the environment is an area of concern. She plans to gather statistics about the population, based on density theories of Rosow,[12] Ardrey,[10] and Freeman.[13]

Fig. 4.8 shows the decision pathway used to arrive at the demographic focus.

Situation B—One of Meg's (P.H.N.) families in her caseload is that of Mr. and Mrs. Smith and their teen-age children. Mr. Smith is unemployed and has been so for several months. Mrs. Smith works part time as a housekeeper. Chris is 17 and a junior in high school; John is 16, a sophomore; and Rudy is 13, and in the eighth grade.

General grand tour	Observation of family behavior.
	Nurse's observations: Each member of the family is so preoccupied with his own troubles that he is unable to offer support and encouragement to the other members.
Social/Cultural system	
	Family Response: Meg checks with each family member. Mr. Smith confirms that he is depressed and spends long hours alone watching television. Mrs. Smith is frustrated and feels "put-down" with her employment. Chris has one boyfriend after another and goes through a deep depression after each friendship ends. John is upset because he doesn't have money for the recreational activities common to his peers. Rudy is an overly active child who demands frequent attention and money for recreational activities. He gets neither.

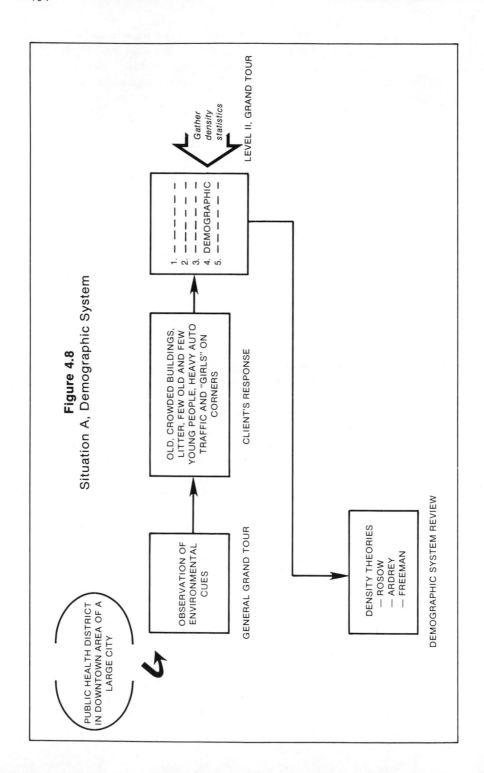

Figure 4.8
Situation A, Demographic System

> Analysis: Meg concludes from her observations
> and the family's responses that the family as
> a social/cultural environment is in trouble.
> She will continue her assessment based on
> Ardrey's social/cultural theory[10] and Sumner's
> ethnocentric theory.[14]

The logic used in assessing the Smith family and arriving at a social/cultural concern is summarized in fig. 4.9.

In each of the prior situations an algorithm process for focusing the assessment has been illustrated. In each case the nurse concludes the initial assessment by formulating a nursing diagnosis(es) with subsequent implementation of a plan of care. All these phases will be documented in nursing histories, care plans, charts, or survey reports.

ASSESSMENT AND DOCUMENTATION: FOUR CASE STUDIES

The next four case studies present clients in three different settings. The settings, to a certain extent, dictate the most likely systems that require immediate assessment. For example, in an emergency or intensive-care setting there are likely to be clients whose physiological needs are paramount. General acute care suggests the likelihood of physical needs, as well as need for care of any or all the remaining systems of man. Of necessity, in extended care and in the community, all Man's systems should probably be assessed. A starting point may be the overt presenting problem, keeping in mind that one must ascertain the client's preception of what is most important, or of greatest concern. With respect to documentation, nursing histories, care plans, and progress notes are shown.

Case Study 1

Donald West, R.N., a community-health nurse, receives a referral form containing the following information:

Name: Bobbie Hardy
Address: 000 Risk Road

Reason for Referral: Bobbie, age 7, has high absenteeism from
   school. Records reveal that he has cerebral palsy and is
   prone to frequent respiratory infections. Unable to contact
   mother. Mother works at Circle K coffee shop on 4th Street.

Person Making Referral: Mr. Benjamin, school counselor.

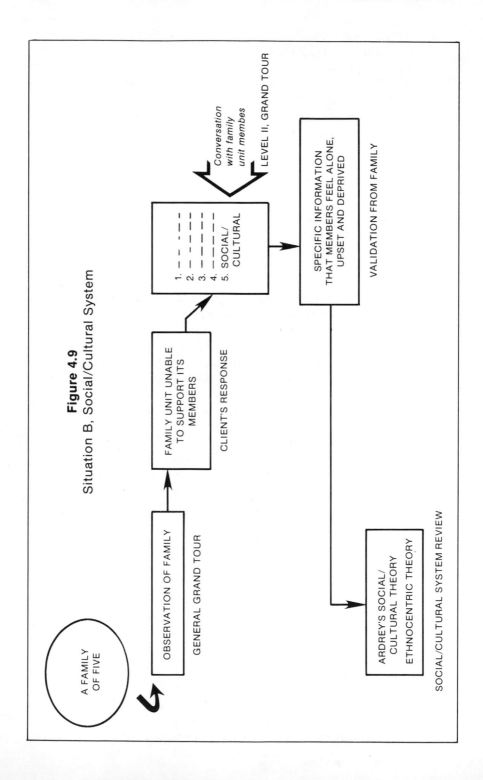

Figure 4.9
Situation B, Social/Cultural System

The nurse phones the coffee shop to make an appointment with Mrs. Hardy. A meeting is set up for her day off next week — 4:00 PM on Tuesday. Donald West, the nurse, uses a client-centered approach in his practice. This means that even though the referral mentions a presenting problem, Donald will identify the client's perception of the situation through grand-tour questions and observations.

The nurse and Mrs. Hardy are together.

Nurse: "How do things seem to be going for you?"

Mrs. Hardy: "We're making it somehow, but it's getting harder all the time."

Nurse: Nods head and listens.

Mrs. Hardy: "I'm surprised you came to see me about Bobbie. He's not my problem. It's Tom Jr. — he's about to drive me crazy. I don't know what he's going to do from one minute to the next. I'm really worried about him; I think he's running around with a group of kids who use drugs and he won't talk to me any more. He stays out too late on school nights. His grades are terrible, but I know he can do better. I know he really needs a father. I'm afraid of what's going to happen! He's already been picked up by the police once."

Nurse: "So its Tom Jr. who's really a concern to you right now?"

Mrs. Hardy: "Well — I guess so. The baby's doing all right. And even though Bobbie's missed a little school, Easter Seals really help out. Cindi — well — she's had a few boyfriend problems but I'm used to that. She's always been a little moody."

Analysis: Nurse Don West has asked his first grand-tour question and as a result has gained clues about Mrs. Hardy's perception of her situation. At this point it seems clear that Tom Jr. is the focus of her concern. The nurse validates his perception of the situation by asking a second grand-tour question. Clues offered by Mrs. Hardy suggest that her concerns relate to the interactive/affiliative system of man.

Nurse: "Is anyone able to help you with your concerns about Tom?"

Mrs. Hardy: "No, I don't know where to turn. His dad's been gone for three years — I don't know where he is. My parents live across the country. They'd help me if they could but they have enough problems of their own. I really don't know what he needs because he won't talk to me. I just feel helpless. In fact, if I didn't have to worry about him, I think I could cope."

Analysis: The nurse has received validation that Tom Jr.'s situation is the mother's greatest concern. The nurse now has two choices. He can pursue specific questions relative to the interactive/affiliative system with the mother or he can choose to assess Tom's perception of the situation. The nurse chooses to talk to Tom directly, securing permission from Tom's mother to do so.

Subsequently, the nurse makes an appointment to meet Tom at a place and time of Tom's choosing. He agrees.

Nurse: "Why did you decide to come here and talk with me today?"

Tom Jr.:   "I was curious. What do you want me for?"

Nurse: "Your mom said you were having some problems. I just wanted to see what you thought about it."

Tom Jr.:   "I miss my friends, we had to move to this dump and school's awful. I don't even have a room of my own anymore. There's nothing to do but hang around with the guys."

Analysis: The nurse can now pursue the questions under the interactive/affiliative system. The questions need not be asked as specifically phrased, but the main thought of each question is used.

Table 4.3 (p. 152) shows the completed assessment guide for Tom Jr.'s situation.

Having completed the interview, it is necessary for the nurse to validate his perceptions with Tom Jr. (shown in Table 4.3). It will be noticed that Tom disagreed with several inferences. These should be reevaluated on a subsequent assessment. Meanwhile, those inferences that are validated become documented as nursing diagnoses for the planning process.

Documenting the Planning Process

Having formulated the nursing diagnoses, the nurse, in collaboration with Tom Jr., will establish behavior or situations he would like to achieve (expected outcomes) and formulate those actions necessary to achieve such behavior (nursing orders). Documentation of the collaborative plan as articulated by the nurse is illustrated in Fig. 4.10.

Problem-Oriented Charting — Case Study 1

Further documentation of Tom Jr.'s status is shown in the following charts, using the problem-oriented method. Because the assessment guide and care plan have already been written, the following illustration shows only the problem list and progress notes.

Problem List

Active Problems   Inactive Problems

3/6 1. Anxious due to change in self-
image and role perception.
D. West, R.N.

3/6 2. Uncertainty due to loss of control
over life-style changes.
D. West, R.N.

3/6 3. Identity crisis due to loss of
father and old friends.
D. West, R.N.

4/6 4. Experiencing conflict due to
demands of family responsibilities and
those of establishing a new friendship.
D. West, R.N.

Initial Plan

1. Anxiety due to change in self-image and role perception.

Diagnostic Plans:	Investigate other sources for peer socialization.
	Explore potential "Big Brother" type relationships.
Therapeutic Plans:	Help Tom identify peers who have similar values.
	Explore feelings about Mom.
Patient-Education Plans:	Discuss normal feelings for age.

2. Uncertainty due to loss of control over life-style changes.

Diagnostic Plans:	Investigate potential areas of control.

Therapeutic Plans: Reflective listening.
Patient-Education Plans: Discuss need to maintain some control and realistic expectations for age.

3. Identity crisis due to loss of father and old friends.

Diagnostic Plans: Explore possibility of reestablishing contact with old friends.
Therapeutic Plans: Explore feelings about father.
Patient-Education Plans: Discuss family structure and his place, role, and expectations.

D. West, R.N.

Progress Notes

DATE	NO.	PROBLEM	PROGRESS NOTES
3/6	See Nursing History and Initial Plan.		
4/6	1,	Anxious due to chg. in self-image and role perception.	S— I've found a neat guy at the Y. He likes to swim and play tennis. He doesn't have a Dad either. O—Animated when talking about new friend. A—Behavior indicates more positive feelings about self. P—Continue previous plan.
4/6	2.	Uncertainty due to loss of control over life style changes.	S— Nothing's changed at home. School is still pretty awful. O— A—Still unable to identify areas of control. P—Continue previous plan.

DATE	NO.	PROBLEM	PROGRESS NOTES
4/6	3.	Identity crisis due to loss of father and old friends.	S— I don't think I want to call my old friends. Jimmy's uncle has been taking us out to play tennis, though. O—Enthusiastic; relaxed when discussing old friends. A— Establishing a potentially meaningful friendship with peer. Seems to be seeking a father image. Has not yet expressed feelings about own father. P— Continue previous plan except delete possibility of contacting old friends.

At the time of the third visit, the nurse reexplored the inferences that had been made during the initial assessment. Tom Jr. now agrees that he is experiencing some conflict between what his mother wants and expects him to do (take care of younger brother) and the expectations of his new-found friend. For this reason, the nurse adds a fourth problem to the problem list.

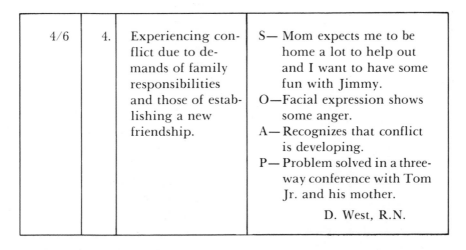

| 4/6 | 4. | Experiencing conflict due to demands of family responsibilities and those of establishing a new friendship. | S— Mom expects me to be home a lot to help out and I want to have some fun with Jimmy.
 O—Facial expression shows some anger.
 A— Recognizes that conflict is developing.
 P— Problem solved in a three-way conference with Tom Jr. and his mother.
 D. West, R.N. |

Mr. West continues to see Tom at the planned two-week intervals. Tom continues to make progress toward solving his problems. The nurse's complete interim progress notes are not shown here but would continue to document his progress. Meanwhile Mr. West has conferred with Mrs. Hardy and has completed an assessment of her and the remaining children. For the purposes of illustration, Tom Jr.'s discharge note is shown below.

			PROGRESS NOTES
DATE	NO.	PROBLEM	PROGRESS NOTES

DISCHARGE SUMMARY

DATE	NO.	PROBLEM	PROGRESS NOTES
6/6	1.	Anxiety	S— Jimmy and I are good friends now. We even found another guy who's okay too. O—Animated — seems self-assured when discussing friendship. A— Problem resolving satisfactorily. P— No further follow-up.
6/6	2.	Uncertainty	S— I guess school will never change but I can manage. Mom helped me turn a corner of the bedroom into my area. My brothers aren't allowed to enter that area unless I say it's okay. O—Seems not happy but accepting of current status. A— Problem resolving satisfactorily considering circumstances. P— Refer mother to social worker to determine eligibility for a larger apartment (3-bedroom).
6/6	3.	Identity crisis...	S— I still don't understand why my Dad left us. I would like to see him

DATE	NO.	PROBLEM	PROGRESS NOTES
			again though. I like to do things with Jimmy's uncle but I still wish Dad were back. O—Appears angry. A—Beginning to verbalize feelings about father. Has established a stable friendship with a peer and a father image. P—No further follow-up.
6/6	4.	Experience of conflict	S—Cindi and I have worked out a plan with Mom so we know what we have to do and when we're free. O— A—Appears satisfied with current plan. P—No further follow-up. Close to service. D. West, R.N.

Case Study 2

Heather, 19 years old, transferred to the orthopedic unit after two weeks in ICU recovering from an injury suffered in a skiing accident. Her physical condition is stable. She is immobilized on a rotating bed. Cervical traction is in place, attached to crutchfield tongs. Jody Sharp, R.N. has chosen to act as her primary nurse.

Jody is performing her initial assessment and begins by asking Heather the following grand-tour question:

Jody: "How are things going for you, Heather?"

Heather: "I just want to get up and move around. I'm sick of lying in this bed. I hope that I won't have to lie still much longer."

Jody: (To verify her perceptions, asks the following grand-tour question)
            "So it is the activity restriction that's really bothering you right now?"

Figure 4.10
Care Plan for Tom Jr.

STANDARDS FOR DISCHARGE OR MAINTENANCE: 3/6 Establishes social contacts with peers
4/6 Resolves family conflicts.   D. West, R.N.

DATE	PROBLEMS	EXPECTED OUTCOMES	DEADLINES	NURSING ORDERS	COMPLETED
3/6	Anxiety due to change in self-image and role perceptions.	Verbalizes better feelings about self in relationship to peers.	3 mos. 6/6 $\sqrt{q}$ 2 wks.	Help Tom identify peers within school setting who have similar values. Investigate other sources for peer socialization. Explore potential "Big Brother" type relationships. Explore feelings about Mom — why have they changed.	
3/6	Uncertainty due to loss of control over life-style changes.	Identifies an area of control.	3 mos. 6/6 $\sqrt{q}$ 2 wks.	At each visit, spend some time investigating potential areas of control.	
3/6	Identity crisis due to loss of father and old friends.	Verbalizes both feelings and perceptions of why father left.	3 mos. 6/6 $\sqrt{q}$ 2 wks.	Explore feelings about father.	

					D/C 4/6
4/6	Experience of conflict due to demands of family responsibilities and those of establishing a new friendship.*	Identifies a friendship group or person.		Explore possibility of re-establishing contact with old friends. See first set of Nursing Orders D. West, R.N.	
		Verbalizes feasible ways of meeting mother's expectations and still having time for friend.	2 mos. 6/6 √ q̄ 2 wks.	Problem-solve in a three-way conference with Tom Jr. and mother.	
		Mother expresses willingness to assist him plan for meeting his various obligations & wishes.		Help both to evaluate how well their plan is working. D. West, R.N.	

*On 4/6 nurse added a diagnosis that was originally not validated by Tom Jr. By 4/6 he could agree that this was a concern.

166

Heather: "I'm tired of a lot of things but I really can't stand to lie still, hooked up to this rope. It's just not me to be this way. I can't do anything. I even have to read upside down."

> Analysis: The second grand-tour question has elicited a response which verifies the nurse's perception that the mobility system of man is a primary focus. Specific observations and questions relative to the mobility system ensue. For the purposes of this illustration, Barsch's Theory of Mobility:
> Movement is one of three critical capabilities for Man's survival[11]
> is the basis for assessment. The physical system of man will not be included nor will assessment based on systems theory and cultural theory. This illustration represents an incomplete assessment of Heather. Total assessment would include all systems of man.

Table 4.4 (p. 188) shows the completed nursing assessment guide which results from Jody's assessment of Heather. Questions, when posed to Heather, were not phrased exactly as written on the form, but adapted to the client situation.

Documenting the Planning Process

Fig. 4.11 shows the care plan for Heather relative to the one nursing diagnosis which resulted from a partial assessment of the mobility system.

Outcome-Oriented Charting — Case Study 2

Jody, the nurse, is utilizing the outcome-oriented method of charting. The assessment guide and care plan comprise the first elements of her documentation and are part of the permanent record. Her charting is shown on the progress notes and care plan.

DATE	PROGRESS NOTES
ADMISSION 2/10 4 P.M.	Admitted at 4 P.M. to room 412. Total systems review completed. See nursing history and care plan. J. Sharp, R.N.
INTERIM 2/11 9 P.M.	States she's glad to be able to watch television when she wants to, and to be able to call home and friends. Demonstrates correct use of bed control. Able to

	relate how bed functions. States she'd still like to get out of the room: "It's really drab." J. Sharp, R.N.
2/13 6 P.M.	Spent one hour in lounge — conversing and dining with friends. States she feels super! J. Sharp, R.N.

Heather continues to progress satisfactorily. Traction is changed from skeletal to skin and she is transferred from the rotating bed to a standard orthopedic bed. As she improves physically, she becomes progressively more mobile and less frustrated. Her room is gaily decorated and she is assertive and spontaneous in her interactions with friends and staff, already thinking ahead to her next ski trip. Jody, the primary nurse, is responsible for Heather's care the entire time, and updates the care plan at appropriate intervals. On 2/17, she formulates a standard for discharge which is shown in the Fig. 4.11. The discharge summary as written on the chart is shown below.

DATE	*PROGRESS NOTES*
DISCHARGE SUMMARY 3/12	Has applied own cervical collar correctly for the last three days. Verbalizes confidence in applying collar at home. Has ambulated around the unit, using normal means of expression — gesturing. Has identified she can participate within range of limited movement and safety. Discharge ambulatory with cervical collar in place. J Sharp, R.N.

Figure 4.11
Care Plan for Heather

STANDARDS FOR DISCHARGE OR MAINTENANCE: *2/10 Deferred for one week (2/17). J.S., R.N. 2/17 Demonstrates safe ambulation techniques with neck collar. Making plans to resume leisure activities within safe limits. J.S., R.N.*

DATE	PROBLEMS	EXPECTED OUTCOMES	DEADLINES	NURSING ORDERS	COMPLETED
2/10	Extremely frustrated due to restricted movement and associated loss of control over activities.	Verbalizes reduced frustration as a result of being able to manipulate environment.	2/13/78 P.M.	Teach how to use bed control to achieve 45° angle in supine position for watching television.	
		Demonstrates correct use of bed control, ability to use telephone, turn on television, and read by self.	2/13 P.M.	Ask family to bring in portable radio. Place on bedside table within reach.	Done 2/11 J.S.
				Encourage patient, family, and friends to make wall decorations.	Done 2/12 N.Z.
				Obtain prism glasses for use by client.	

		Done 2/11 N.Z.
Obtain touch-tone telephone model, place console with phone within reach.		
Check into policy regarding unit confinement, explore possibility of taking to lounge once/day for stimulation. J. Sharp, R.N.		

Case Study 3

Allistar Rand is a corporate president, 55 years old, divorced, and living alone without an immediate family. About three weeks ago he fell unconscious during a board meeting and was subsequently admitted to an acute-care setting and treated for a cerebral vascular accident. At this time, he has been transferred to a convalescent-care center for an active rehabilitation program. The anticipated length of stay is approximately three weeks. Nurse Ellen Change is ready to conduct an initial assessment of Mr. Rand. She has already completed the physical examination and finds that Mr. Rand has mild expressive aphasia. His sense of touch, vision, hearing, taste, and smell are all essentially intact and functioning. There is generalized weakness and lack of fine motor coordination of the right side of his body. He is able to ambulate with a walker. Muscle size and tone are within norms. Skin is intact with evidence of adequate circulation. The fact that he has mild expressive aphasia leads the nurse to conclude that the sensory/perceptive system of man is one focus for further in-depth assessment. Table 4.5 (p. 190) documents this assessment which resulted in three nursing diagnoses. The care plan is formulated and appears in Fig. 4.12.

The charting policy in the convalescent-care center requires outcome-oriented charting. Ms. Change makes the following initial entry:

> Nursing assessment completed.
> Sensory/perceptive problems identified.
> See nursing history and care plan.
> E. Change, R.N.

Outcome-Oriented Charting — Case Study 3

DATE	PROGRESS NOTES
INTERIM NOTES	
4/19 11 A.M.	Is able to choose among three alternatives in selecting mealtime and menu selection. Initiates other choices at times. J. Power, R.N.
8 P.M.	Beginning to consider ways to live at home and maintain home environment. Making some business decisions via telephone. E. Change, R.N.
4/15 9 P.M.	Performing A.D.L. independently. Actively involved in business communications and dictation. States he has decided to hire a full-time homemaker and will maintain his position as president of the corporation by working from his home at first. E. Change, R.N.

DISCHARGE SUMMARY	
5/2 9 A.M.	Has hired a full-time housekeeper and he states that the corporation board is supportive of his business decision regarding his management position. Expressing confidence in his communication skills and rapid improvement, looking forward to swimming and golfing by summer.
	Discharge ambulatory with correct use of cane, accompanied by two corporate secretaries. J. Power, R.N.

The situations just discussed have arbitrarily represented information that specifically guided the nurse to assess only one system of man. In reality, of course, situations are not singular and pure. They are complicated, and clients move from one setting to another. The complexities of clients' and nurses' real situations require more comprehensive assessments and varieties of documentation than have been previously illustrated. The following narration is designed to depict a "real" situation.

Case Study 4

Mr. Flint was admitted to the coronary intensive-care unit and diagnosed as having a massive coronary occlusion. The situation requires assessment of the physiological system. His diagnosis demands that priority be given to the cardiovascular subsystem of the physiological system. This assessment of the psychological and interactive/affiliative systems of man. continuing basis. Fig. 4.13 shows an example of a flow sheet which might be used.

As Mr. Flint's condition stabilizes, other systems require attention. These may be other subsystems within the physiological system, as well as some of the other systems of man. In the case of Mr. Flint, it has been determined that he is 36 years old and is a career military pilot, flying experimental jets. He is married, with one daughter who is three years old. Interactions with the patient and the family reveal many problems that require further assessment of the sensory/perceptive and mobility systems. The intensive-care environment and the enforced restriction of activity of a previously very active person precipitate problems causing further assessment of the sensory/perceptive and mobility system. The nursing diagnoses deduced from these assessments result in care plans, progress notes, and continuing flow sheets consistent with the theories associated with these several systems.

Figure 4.12
Care Plan for Mr. Rand

STANDARDS FOR DISCHARGE OR MAINTENANCE: *4/12 Articulates realistic plans for resuming life-style consistent with his values.   E. Change, R.N.*

DATE	PROBLEMS	EXPECTED OUTCOMES	DEADLINES	NURSING ORDERS	COMPLETED
4/12	Extremely frustrated due to inability to name objects and organize thoughts.	Consistently and correctly names common objects. Verbalizes that thought disorganization is typical of a stroke and will resolve. Converses understandably, socially, and with business associates on phone.	5/2 √ q̄ day A.M.	Talk as with anyone who understands. Engage him in a conversation that requires serial content at least 2x daily. If frustration develops, use gestures rather than repeating word instructions. Practice naming by pointing to objects and clearly enunciating their names. Encourage him to repeat words after you. Pace speech to his responses.	
4/12	Inability to make independent choices due to interrupted though patterns.	Makes simple choices regarding activities of daily living. Identifies alternatives regarding life style.	4/19 √ q̄ day A.M. 4/25 √ q̄ day P.M.	Allow choices regarding A.D.L. as much as possible. Practice problem-solving skills, considering alternatives, daily.	

Date		Date	
4/12	Anger due to conflict between perceived current self-image and preferred self-image.		
	Performs A.D.L. independently. Engages in business conversations and decisions. Verbalizes ways to maintain preferred personal style. Verbalizes that he is feeling okay about himself.	4/25 √q̄ day P.M.	Discuss future goals or plans on an ongoing basis. Delegate to E. Change, R.N. Allow independence even if slow. Encourage participation in business. Discuss personal life-style preferences and problem-solve achieving them. Active & reflective listening for feelings content. E. Change, R.N.

Figure 4.13
Flow Sheet, Coronary Occlusion

CLINICAL PARAMETERS	PATIENT OUTCOME PROFILE									
DX: Coronary Occlusion	HOURLY TIME FRAMES									
Chest Pain										
Perspiration										
Weakness										
Apprehension										
Restlessness										
Dizziness										
Dyspnea										
Orthopnea										
Coughing/Sneezing										
Nausea/Vomiting										
Abdominal Bloating										
EKG:										
Q-Waves										
↑ S.T.										
T-Waves										
Apical Pulse										
Heart Sounds										
Lung Sounds										
Response to Analgesic										

(This flow sheet is an example only — not intended to represent a comprehensive assessment)

After three weeks, Mr. Flint is transferred out of the coronary care unit to the medical unit. The care plan that accompanies him on transfer documents those problems still present in the systems previously assessed. The primary nurse on the medical unit becomes aware, at this point in Mr. Flint's convalescence, of many learning needs which lead to a detailed assessment of the cognitive/intellectual system. Meanwhile, assessments of the wife and daughter, nursing diagnoses, and plans have also been included in the total nursing process and its documentation. One of the results of the cognitive/intellectual assessment is implementation of the standard teaching plan for myocardial infarction patients.

An environmental assessment was initiated by the primary nurse through referral to the discharge planner. This assessment took place in the home to identify potential problems (or lack of problems) in the physical and mobility environmental systems. Findings, in conjunction with those of the ongoing assessment of the primary nurse, uncovered problems in the home environment. The home is two-storied, with upstairs bedrooms. The wife works outside of the home eight to ten hours a day and has a babysitter for the three-year-old child at home. For these and other reasons, more in-depth assessments were made relative to all the environmental systems.

This total assessment resulted in a referral to a community health nurse for ongoing post-discharge care. Some environmental adaptations were made. The downstairs den was converted into a bedroom; the three-year-old was enrolled in a nursery school; and a part-time homemaker was hired to care for the home and prepare a special diet.

Several months went by without substantial improvement in Mr. Flint's cardiac status. His special diet, limited tolerance for activity, and psychological problems associated with changes in self-image and role in family resulted in conclusions by the community health nurse that a complete assessment of all systems of man was necessary. Problems were identified relative to Maslow's hierarchy of needs,[15] Peplau's theory of anxiety,[3] Neugarten and Birren's theory of mastery and competence,[16,17] Festinger's theory of cognitive dissonance,[6] Angyal's intimacy theory,[18] Sarbin's role theory[9], Erickson's theory of psychological growth and development[19], Ardrey's theory of personal space[10], and Barsch's theory of movement,[11] including biological rhythms. All these problems were not unique to Mr. Flint but encompassed the family as a client.

Documentation of the assessments, nursing diagnoses, plans of care, and client responses were accomplished in several ways throughout the entire episode. In the coronary care unit, progress notes took the form of flow sheets and outcome-oriented narratives. On the medical unit, outcome-oriented charting predominated (consistent with agency policy), and in the home setting, the community nurse utilized the problem-oriented method.

Table 4.1
Level II Grand-Tour Questions: Man

SYSTEMS OF MAN	THEMES	LEVEL TWO GRAND TOUR (OBSERVATIONS AND QUESTIONS)
Physiological	Vital signs Pain Dysfunction or displacement of body part	Can you tell me more specifically about it? Can you describe how you felt? How long have you felt this way? Have you felt this way before? *If these questions elicit responses of significant concern, refer to pages 225-286 for more detailed assessment standards and questions.*
Psychological	Interest Enjoyment Satisfaction Progressive growth and development	Respond to the non-verbal cues that client presents. Pick up on emphasized words or ideas. When you talk or think about this, where do you feel it in your body? More specifically, what seems to be happening? *If these questions elicit responses of significant concern, refer to pages 288-293 for more detailed assessment standards and questions.*
Cognitive/Intellectual	Self-awareness Selectivity Control of environment Mastery Competence Wide array of cognitive skills	How do you feel about what is happening to you? How are you able to handle this situation? *If these questions elicit responses of significant concern, refer to pages 295-297 for more detailed assessment standards and questions.*

		Skills to achieve own ends Control of impulses	
Sensory/Perceptive	Ability to understand Perception of meanings Perception of self Perception of alternatives Values	Has anything like this happened before? Do you understand what is happening to you? How do you feel about yourself right now? What choices or alternatives seem available? *If these questions elicit responses of significant concern, refer to pages 300-302 for more detailed assessment standards and questions.*
Interactive/Affiliative	Coping with environment Satisfactory feedback from others Closeness with another Affecting or being affected by others Reference/support groups Roles Personal space	How are others affecting you right now? How is your situation affecting you at this time? Is anyone able to help you in this situation? *If these questions elicit responses of significant concern, refer to pages 304-308 for more detailed assessment standards and questions.*
Mobility	Dynamic balance (physical) Body schema Spacial awareness Orientation to time Life rhythms	Are you able to move about in order to accomplish what you need to do? Does time seem to be going faster or slower right now? Are you able to maintain your normal routines? *If these questions elicit responses of significant concern, refer to pages 310-312 for more detailed assessment standards and questions.*

Table 4.1 *(cont.)*
Level II Grand-Tour Questions: Man

SYSTEMS OF MAN	THEMES	LEVEL TWO GRAND TOUR (OBSERVATIONS AND QUESTIONS)
Economic	Standard of living	In what ways: Are you satisfied with your current standard of living? Has your standard of living changed? Is your standard of living meeting your needs. *If these questions elicit responses of significant concern, refer to page 317 for more detailed assessment standards and questions.*
Physical	Inefficiency Irritability Proneness to illness or accidents Allergy	Do you feel that your environment is safe? What has happened, or might happen? Can you describe what is bothering you? *If these questions elicit responses of significant concern, refer to pages 319-325 for more detailed assessment standards and questions.*
Mobile	Freedom of physical and social movement Goal fulfillment Attachment, involvement, and satisfaction	Are you able to move about as you desire? Do you have any problems with your transportation? Are you as close as you would like to be with people of you choice? *If these questions elicit responses of significant concern, refer to page 327 for more detailed assessment standards and questions.*

| Demographic | Morale
Satisfactory amount of social awareness
Right amount of necessities and amenities
Conformance or violence | Are you satisfied with your housing situation?
How about you neighbors?
  Right number of them
  Not too dependent
  Not too violent
  Not too isolated
What kinds of resources (money, services, cultural experiences, entertainment) are available to you?
If these questions elicit responses of significant concern, refer to page 329 for more detailed assessment standards and questions. |
| Social/Cultural | Opportunity for identity, stimulation, and security
"Own" referent group
Learned ways of thinking and acting | Have your ideas about yourself changed?
Are your beliefs or values pretty consistent with those of your friends and neighbors?
How secure do you feel in your present situation?
How stimulating is your environment?
How do you feel about yourself right now?
If these questions elicit responses of significant concern, refer to pages 331-332 for more detailed assessment standards and questions. |

Table 4.2
Level II Grand-Tour Questions: Environment*

SYSTEMS OF MAN	THEMES	LEVEL TWO GRAND TOUR (OBSERVATIONS AND QUESTIONS)

Economic	Supply and demand
	Manpower
	Land
	Liquid capital
	Technology
	System of exchange
	Units of barter
		For a specific area — what is general standard of living
		    low
		    medium
		    high?

Physical	Comfort or safety:
	    air
	    water
	    noise
	    temperature
	    radiation
	    chemical
	    microbiol
	    hazards, safety
		Obtain general statistics regarding factors.

Mobile	Communication systems Transit systems Group networks	Observe for means of or plans for communication and mobility. If preliminary information suggests inadequate mobility systems, see page 327.

Demographic	Density	Observe for density and characteristics of population.
	Growth-rate trend	
	Death-rate trend	
	Presymptomatic illness trends	
	Special risk groups	
	Overcrowding or undercrowding	
Social/Cultural	Individual and group stimuli	Observe for social and cultural norms.
	Cultural habits	
	Security	

*Level Two Grand-Tour questions as shown in this table are designed to be used as screening questions only. If a screening question reveals a problem, the nurse refers to an environmental specialist.

Table 4.3

Interactive/Affiliative System: Assessment Guide — Tom, Jr.

- Interpersonal Theories

STANDARD 1. Presence of feelings of security in most important interpersonal relationships.	INFERENCES Met Not Met √	VALIDATION Agreed √ Disagreed	NURSING DIAGNOSIS (DEDUCTION) Anxious due to change in self-image and role perception.
Questions, Observations, Examinations			Client's Responses
1. How do you feel about what is happening to you? Put down Not recognized or valued			"Mad"
2. Do you feel you have control over what is happening to you?			No — I didn't want to move. I don't know why my Dad left us.
3. Has something like this ever happened before; what do you remember about it?			No — before Dad left everything was great.
4. Who, if anyone, can help (be supportive of you) at this time?			Nobody — the kids pick on me because I'm different than they are: I just don't like to do what they do.
5. Who are the important people in your life? family significant others work group social group			I don't know. I just hang around with some guys who come over from the other side of town. Dad would know what to do.

6. Do relationships with these people make you feel comfortable/uncomfortable?

    now

    past

    potential in future

No — but I had to prove myself to the guys. I'm no sissy. All my good buddies are back where we used to live.

7. What interactions, if any, tend to upset you?

Mom — she keeps bugging me. The kids at school won't leave me alone and neither will my brothers.

- Observations

    Body language

    Posture

    Muscle tension

    Facial expressions

    Random/compulsive movements

    Tone of voice

Fidgety

Rigid posture

Mixture — almost on verge of tears, yet trying to put on a brave front.

Range — from strong intensity to nonchalance

- Communication Theories

	INFERENCES		NURSING DIAGNOSES (DEDUCTIONS)
STANDARD 2. Able to change behavior of self or others in an attempt to reduce anxiety.	Met Not Met √	VALIDATION Agreed √ Disagreed	*Uncertain due to loss of control over life-style changes.*
STANDARD 3. Able to communicate in interpersonal and group relationships.	Met √ Not Met	Agreed √ Disagreed	

Table 4.3 *(cont.)*

Interactive/Affiliative System: Assessment Guide — Tom, Jr.

Questions, Observations, Examinations	Client's Responses
8. How do you usually find out what others expect of you?	*Oh — my mother lets me know.*
9. How easy or difficult is it for you to follow through?	*Why bother — where does it get you?*
10. In your past how have you been able to respond to your own or others' expectations?	*It was, oh, when Dad was here. I was one of the group before.*
11. Do you usually feel in control of the situation or a victim of the circumstances?	*See question 2.*
12. How have you generally responded to pressures for change in your life style?	*I hate it — I don't have any fun anymore.*
13. What type of work do you do?	*Go to school. I have to babysit with Johnnie.*
14. How do you spend your leisure time?	*Hanging around. I like to swim but we don't have a pool anymore.*
15. How do you feel about your achievements in life?	*I used to be on the honor roll and I was pretty good at tennis too. I won a trophy one time.*
16. What important things do you feel you have accomplished?	*See question 15.*

• Observations
    Transmitting ideas clearly.
    Receiving or understanding.
    Validating or checking out.
	Communicates clearly.

• Group/Role Theories

	INFERENCES	VALIDATION	NURSING DIAGNOSES (DEDUCTIONS)
STANDARD 4. Membership in one or more social groups.	Met ✓ / Not Met	Agreed ✓ / Disagreed	
STANDARD 5. Membership in a kin network.	Met ✓ / Not Met	Agreed ✓ / Disagreed	
STANDARD 6. Perceived sense of comfort with values and norms of reference groups.	Met / Not Met ✓ *Uncomfortable with family and "guys", due to radical change in values from prior friendship group.*	Agreed / Disagreed ✓ *Tom disagrees; says he feels comfortable with the "group."*	*Inference not substantiated by client.*
STANDARD 7. Able to rank loyalties among reference groups.	Met / Not Met ✓ *Conflict between demands of family and "guys."*	Agreed / Disagreed ✓ *Says it isn't a problem.*	*Inference not substantiated by client.*
STANDARD 8. Satisfaction with role identity.	Met / Not Met ✓	Agreed ✓ / Disagreed	*Identity crisis due to loss of father and old friends.*

Table 4.3 *(cont.)*

Interactive/Affiliative System: Assessment Guide — Tom, Jr.

Questions, Observations, Examinations	Client's Responses
17. Is there someone/s on whom you rely?	*I can take care of myself.*
18. How easy is it to keep in touch with those who are important to you?	*Well, I don't even know where my Dad is. He doesn't need to come back now. Mom better not ever get married again.*
19. What groups are you affiliated with?	*The guys — see question 5.*
20. Which do you feel most comfortable with?	*The guys.*
21. How consistent are your opinions and feelings with those in the group?	*See questions 4 through 6.*
22. Which groups are the most important to you?	*My old friends.*
23. How able are you to meet their expectations?	*I was okay with them. I was one of them.*
24. How many roles do you assume right now in your life?	*Big brother — babysitter*
	Student
	Son
	One of the guys
25. Which role is most important?	*One of the guys.*
26. Are you satisfied with this role?	*No.*
• Observations	
Body Language	
Posture	*Rigid*
Muscle tension	
Facial expressions	

Random/compulsive movements
Tone of voice

One of depression
Fidgety

• Intimacy Theories

	INFERENCES	VALIDATION	NURSING DIAGNOSES (DEDUCTION)
STANDARD 9. Closeness with another throughout life.	Met Not Met √ *Suffering from loss of father.*	Agreed Disagreed √ Says, "I don't need my Dad — I can take care of myself."	*Inference not validated by client.*

Questions, Observations, Examinations		Client's Responses
21. What about close personal relationships in your life?		*Dad and I were buddies. We used to go fishing.* *Mom used to be okay when we were a real family.*

• Cultural Theories

	INFERENCES	VALIDATION	NURSING DIAGNOSES (DEDUCTION)
STANDARD 10. A state of being consistent with the values, norms, and goals of the most important reference groups.	Met Not Met √	Agreed Disagreed √ *Refer to Standards 6 and 7.*	Inference not substantiated by client.

Questions, Cues, Inspections		Client's Responses
Refer back to previous questions related to group/role.		

Table 4.4

Mobile System: Assessment Guide — Heather

- Systems Theories

| STANDARD 1. Adequate space in which to exercise movement and express self through gestures, mannerisms, and leisure activities. | INFERENCES
Met
Not Met √ | VALIDATION
Agreed √
Disagreed | NURSING
DIAGNOSIS
(DEDUCTION)

Extremely frustrated due to restricted movement and associated loss of control over activities. |

Questions, Observations, Examinations	Client's Responses
1. Are you used to being an active person?	*Oh yes! I ski every weekend, always doing something — dancing, biking — I can't sit still (grimaces).*
2. Do you have access to transportation? How do you move about your home and community?	*(Not applicable to ask)*
3. Are you able to move about enough to accomplish what you need to?	*With help I can brush my teeth and wash my face. Actually, I can't do anything for myself unless someone helps me.*
4. Are you able to move about enough to accomplish those things you like to do?	*I really can't stand to lie still hooked up to this rope — it's just not me.*
5. How do you express your feelings through movement?	*I gesture a lot — move my head and body. When I'm upset I take long walks.*

• Observations
  Obstacles to movement.
  Stimuli for movement (colors, patterns, sounds, other people)
  Policies that affect movement.

  Social norms that affect movement.
  Transportation systems (wheelchairs, crutches, public, car, body power).

In traction, crutchfield tongs. Private room, light green walls, gray floors, white curtains. One picture behind bed — set operational.
Visiting hours limited to one hour in afternoon and evening. Against rules for patient to leave unit.

Movable, rotating bed.

Table 4.5

Sensory Perceptive System: Assessment Guide — Mr. Rand

Perception Theories	INFERENCES	VALIDATION	NURSING DIAGNOSES (DEDUCTIONS)
STANDARD 1. Presence of intact sensory receptors.	Met √ Not Met	Agreed √ Disagreed	
STANDARD 2. Ability to recall consequential facts or events.	Met √ Not Met	Agreed √ Disagreed	
STANDARD 3. Selective responses to stimuli that are consistent with the environment and organism itself.	Met √ Not Met	Agreed √ Disagreed	
STANDARD 4. Ability to organize and label events, objects, and situations.	Met Not Met √	Agreed √ Disagreed	*Extremely frustrated due to inability to name objects and organize thoughts.*
STANDARD 5. Ability to predict consequences of a situation based on previous and current perceptions.	Met Not Met √	Agreed √ Disagreed	*Inability to make independent choices due to interrupted thought patterns.*
STANDARD 6. Behavior consistent with own values.	Met Not Met √	Agreed √ Disagreed	*Anger due to conflict between perceived current self-image and preferred self-image.*

Questions, Observations, Examinations	Client's Responses
1. Has anything like this happened to you before? If yes, how did you respond to the last time?	*Not applicable*
2. How is the situation similar or different to what happened before?	*Not applicable*
3. Do you know anyone else that this has happened to?	*Yes, but I never thought it would happen to me. John had the same trouble two years ago. He can't walk right. My father died, fortunately he lived for only a few hours after it happened to him.*
Perform objective exam for labeling objects.	*Determined by examination: Unable to name telephone, water glass, briefcase, pen. Able to name other objects in room.*
4. What do these symptoms or this situation mean to you?	*Unable to respond with meaningful content and sentences. Could relate that he was having some kind of problem.*
5. How do you feel about what is happening to you?	*It's intolerable. (Observed high tension level at this question — tried to say more — unable to. Began talking about different subjects — unaware of switch.*
6. How does your family feel about what is happening to you or about this situation?	*They don't know.*
7. What choices or alternatives seem available right now?	*Unable at this time to articulate alternatives.*

Table 4.5 *(cont.)*

Sensory Perceptive System: Assessment Guide — Mr. Rand

Questions, Observations, Examinations	Client's Responses
8. How is each alternative likely to work out?	*Not applicable*
• Observe for:	
Ease and rate with which questions are answered.	*Difficulty in answering quickly.*
Coherence and continuity of speech.	*Coherent but at times words and thoughts are scrambled.*
Blocking and interrupted train of thought.	*Evident.*
Meaningless repetition or echoing of words.	*Not present.*
9. How easy or difficult is it for you to participate in this situation right now?	*It's terrible. I'm not used to being dependent. I'm usually in control.*
10. How do you feel about yourself right now?	*I hate what's happening.*
• Observe for:	
Muscular tension.	*Not noted.*
Distracted or random movements.	*Tapping fingers of left hand.*
Anxious facial expressions.	*Face tense.*
Disturbances of thought processes.	*Noted earlier in interview.*
Tone of voice.	*Curt.*

REFERENCES

1. Sutterly D, Donnely G: *Perspectives in Human Development.* Philadelphia, JB Lippincott Co, 1973, p 16.
2. Selye H: *The Stress of Life.* New York, McGraw-Hill Book Co, Inc, 1956, pp. 56, 274.
3. Peplau H: A working definition of anxiety. In Burd S, Marshall M (eds): *Some Clinical Approaches to Psychiatric Nursing.* New York, The Macmillan Co, 1963, pp 323-327.
4. Kubler-Ross E: *On Death and Dying.* New York, The Macmillan Co, 1969.
5. Lewin R: Field theory and learning. In Henry N (ed): *The Forty-First Yearbook of the National Society for the Study of Education, Part II: The Psychology of Learning.* Chicago, The University of Chicago Press, 1942, pp 215-245.
6. Festinger L: *A Theory of Cognitive Dissonance.* Stanford, Calif, Stanford University Press, 1957.
7. Day R: *Perception Through Experience.* London, Methuen and Co, Ltd, 1970.
8. Sullivan H: *A Textbook in Analytic Group Psycho-Therapy.* New York, WW Norton and Co, Inc, 1953.
9. Sarbin T: The scientific status of the mental illness metaphor. In Plog S, Edgerton R (eds): *Changing Perspectives in Mental Illness.* New York, Holt, Reinhart and Winston, 1969, pp 23-24.
10. Ardrey R: *The Social Contract.* New York, Atheneum, 1970, pp 23, 89.
11. Barsch RH: *Achieving Perceptual Motor Efficiency, A Space Oriented Approach to Learning,* Vol. 1. Seattle, Special Child Publications, 1967.
12. Rosow S: Housing and local ties of the aged. *Patterns of Living and Housing of Middle-Aged and Older People: Proceedings of Research Conference.* Washington, DC, Department of Health, Education, and Welfare, 1965, pp 47-57.
13. Freeman R: *Community Health Nursing Practice.* Philadelphia, WB Saunders Co, 1970, pp 254-256.
14. Sumner W: *Folkways.* New York, Ginn, 1906, pp 12-13.
15. Maslow A: *Motivation and Personality.* 2nd ed, New York, Harper and Row, 1974.
16. Neugarten B: The Awareness of Middle Age. In Neugarten B (ed): *Middle Age and Aging.* Chicago, The University of Chicago Press, 1968, pp 93-98.
17. Birren J: Psychological Aspects of Aging: Intellectual Functioning. *Gerontologist* 8:16-19, 1968.
18. Angyal A: *Neurosis and Treatment: A Holistic Theory.* New York, John Wiley and Sons, Inc, 1965.
19. Erickson E: Childhood and Society. 2nd ed, New York, WW Norton, 1963.

BIBLIOGRAPHY

AMOSIST Manual: 6th ed, Houston Tex, Department of the Army, Academy of Health Sciences.

Bertziss A: *Data Structures: Theory and Practice.* New York, Academic Press, 1971.

Korphage R: *Logic and Algorithms: With Application to the Computer and Information Sciences.* New York, John Wiley and Sons, Inc, 1966.

Landa L: *Algorithimization in Learning and Instruction.* Englewood Cliffs, NJ, Educational Technology Publications, 1974.

National Center for Health Services Research. Research Digest Series: *Program Analysis of Physician Extender Algorithm Projects (System Sciences, Inc),* Hyattsville, Md, National Center for Health Services Research, 1977.

Schriber T: *Fundamentals of Flow Charting.* New York, John Wiley and Sons, 1969.

5

Implications for Implementation

REALITY ORIENTATION

Implementation implies orientation to reality. It means putting something to work. It means being practical. How then can theories be put to work? Can assessment guides be made practical or feasible for use in the real world of nurses and clients? Most people enjoy dreaming or fantasizing about an ideal world or universe. A conceptual framework can be someone's fantasy rather than a representation of reality.

And so, in order to face reality and to avoid the disillusionment of a nonfunctional "ivory-towered" conceptual framework, a way to interpret reality becomes a necessity. Chater suggests three terms, that, when defined, help one to climb down from the "ivory tower" and place one's feet on the ground. The setting, the learner or care-giver, and knowledge are the three terms used by Chater.[1]

Setting

"Setting...is intended to convey the entire gamut of social, economic, political, and cultural parameters, both internally at the institutional level as well as externally within the immediate and larger community."[2] Paying attention to the realities in the setting forces individuals to deal with real problems and the constraints within which they must function. Implicit in acknowledging the setting is acceptance of certain constraints over which no control can be exercised.

The nurse can imagine herself as one who, for personal reasons, must live in a certain community and thus must work in the local community hospital. She finds herself assigned to manage a unit of 50 patients on the night shift. Her assistant is not a registered nurse. Such a staffing pattern has prevailed in this setting for many years, possibly because of the nonavailability of registered nurses as well as of the community's expectations and values regarding health care. The nurse may wish to make many changes, but the probability of success is low unless she clearly understands the elements of the setting she cannot change.

It has already been clarified that the conceptual framework here can be equally applicable in a nursing-education curriculum or in a client-care service setting. Some substantial differences in the actual implementation of conceptual frameworks in these two settings must, however, be acknowledged. It is requisite that all nationally accredited educational programs be based upon a conceptual framework and that it can be demonstrated to be operational. Nursing service settings have no such requirements. In the academic world, such terminology as constructs, concepts, and theories are natural. This is not so in a service setting. There the language stresses numbers, dollars, acuities, and values. Language and foci of attention are different from those of academe. Obviously, the setting for practice makes a difference and influences whether or not the nurse has a conceptual framework, and how far she can go in pursuing it.

She should not however, be blinded by the constraints of a setting. It is important also to look for the opportunities and positive expectations (such as resources, learning experiences, and positive values) that the setting offers. Nurses are remiss if they fail to pay attention to what the community needs and offers as part of the nursing environment.

Learner or Care-Provider

The learner or care-provider can be described as one of a group with certain specific characteristics. These characteristics create some realities for the development of the nurse's conceptual framework. If learners tend to come from a community of persons whose motivations, interests, and goals are primarily vocational and job-oriented, nursing realities are quite different than if the goals are self-actualizing and care-oriented. Learner characteristics provide direction for selection of theories relative to learning, motivation, performance, and evaluation. An example of learner characteristics are those which may typify a beginning class of students in an upper-division baccalaureate program. In one program students may tend to have a mean age of 27, approximately 50 percent holding a prior degree, and a grade point of 3.6 and above. These characteristics may represent a trend in classes over a period of time. Such learner characteristics give direction to the faculty in selection of teaching-learning methods, sequencing of courses and learning experiences, and expectations for achievement. By contrast, a faculty makes different plans if learner trends reveal a different type of learner—aged 18 to 26, with no prior college degrees, and with lower grade points. In the nursing-service setting, members of the nursing staff have characteristics that help define what it is reasonable to expect in terms of achieving agency goals and establishing performance objectives.

Knowledge

Knowledge is "...an explicit definition of nursing and the conceptual-ization of nursing practice."[2] Grand statements about nursing ideals are often found in an expressed philosophy. Too often, the learners or performers are completely unaware of the institution's basic philosophy and its implications for their own behavior. Even if they have read a statement of the underlying philosophy, it may be too abstract to be understood and followed. The knowledge needed to make a philosophy operational must be made explicit through the conceptual framework. The term "conceptual framework" may imply the world of the ivory tower. But realistically, only a conceptual tool can make the abstract concrete, can define levels of knowledge and competency, and can clarify assumptions and limitations. The operational implications of a conceptual framework are myriad. In practice, that framework provides a blueprint for direction, cohesiveness, and feedback. Finally, the setting, the learner and care-provider, and her knowledge are interrelated and of equal importance in providing training and service. In fact, that framework becomes the key to keeping doors open between education and service.

With the importance of a conceptual framework for the work world understood, what does the nurse do if she does not possess one? She has several alternatives: She

1. gets a representative sample of her group together and step-by-step deductively develops a conceptual framework, starting with purposes and philosophy and arriving at constructs, concepts, and theories.
2. begins by reviewing conceptual frameworks developed by others, obtaining general commitment to one, and modifying it according to the setting, learners or care-givers, and her definition of nursing.
3. starts assessing her environment and looking for opportunities to incorporate some of the elements of theory-based practice, building inductively toward a conceptual framework.

Assuming that in many cases, particularly in the area of service, the third alternative is the one likely to succeed, certain opportunities are at hand. These opportunities are inherent in the daily nursing activities that can be easily reinforced. Some such activities are those of care-planning, auditing, and assessing.

ADAPTING EXISTING ASSESSMENT AND DOCUMENTATION MODELS

In reality, it is often not clearly evident that most care plans, audit criteria, and assessment models are theory-based. In fact, many are influenced by or derived from the medical model, which is disease-oriented.

In spite of this, however, careful scrutiny shows that nurses probably have theories in mind when they express problems, standards, and questions. According to Argyris, nurses are not alone in this informal use of theories.[3] In fact, it may be the rule rather than the exception to function this way. Achieving sophistication in explaining the basis for a theory is evolutionary in every discipline, and is directly related to the value and support the profession gives to research. What is meant, essentially, is informal research—for example, refining what is available in order to become more theory-oriented.

Standard Care Plans

Standard care plans are widely used in a variety of clinical settings, for various reasons: as references for formulating individualized care plans; as predetermined standards of care for assessment, implementation and documentation; and as sources for audit criteria. Standard care plans tend to be labeled and organized according to established systems of coding (the HICDA, Hospital International Classification of Diseases, adapted for use; the ICDA-8, international classification of diseases, adapted for use; and the DSM-II, diagnostic and standard manual of mental disorders).[4] This is consistent with the traditional medical model and is also done to facilitate easy retrieval of patient audit information by medical records departments. Trends are also developing toward the formulation of an official classification of nursing diagnoses.[5,6] In addition to the medical model, standard care plans are also developed according to nursing diagnoses and classification of nursing services rendered, for example, in community health.

Most of these standard care plans relate primarily to patho-physiological theories[7]; however, problems or nursing diagnoses related to the other systems of man can also be found. For example, a standard care plan for the surgical diagnosis of mastectomy contains many indirect theory-related statements. Fig. 5.1 is a classic example of a diagnosis-specific standard care plan. However, as the nurse studies the plan, she finds it easy to identify theory-related themes in many of the statements. For example, the second problem statement "anxiety and fear due to unknown results," associated with the expected-outcome "verbal and non-verbal expression: 'I can cope with what will happen'" contains criteria that can be derived from several theories. The cognitive/intellectual system of man, the systems theory, Festinger's stress theory, cognitive dissonance, and Peplau's theory of anxiety, all can provide a theoretical basis for this nursing diagnosis and the expected-outcome statement. One can look at other problems and expected-outcome statements on the same standard care plan and identify other theory-based items. Such theories are arbitrarily identified from a conceptual framework. It is not known what theory or empirical basis the authors of the care plan in Fig. 5.1 were using.

Figure 5.1

Diagnosis Specific Standard Care Plan — Radical Mastectomy*

DATE	USUAL PROBLEMS	EXPECTED OUTCOMES	DEADLINES	NURSING ORDERS
	PRE-OP **1. Standard**	1. Standard		1. Standard
	2. Anxiety and fear due to unknown results	2. Verbal and non-verbal expression: "I can cope with what will happen"	pre-op	2A. Listen. Let patient verbalize own feelings, hopes, fears and questions B. If surgery is known to be extensive, demonstrate arm exercises C. One nurse to establish a one-to-one relationship for duration of hospitalization
	EARLY POST-OP **1. Grief due to loss of breast**	1. Verbalize feelings Sleep all night without sleep medications	√ daily	1A. Listen and clarify concerns B. Reply with honesty C. Be direct in encouraging interest in getting up, grooming, self-care, etc.
	2. Potential hypostatic pneumonia due to shallow respiration	2. No respiratory distress Temperature under 101 degrees	√ q 8 hr	2A. Be especially thorough with breathing and coughing exercises

Figure 5.1 *(cont.)*

Diagnosis Specific Standard Care Plan — Radical Mastectomy

DATE	USUAL PROBLEMS	EXPECTED\OUTCOMES	DEADLINES	NURSING ORDERS
				B. Give pain medication before deep breathing and coughing C. Ambulate vigorously and frequently
	LATE POST-OP **1. Limited movement and edema of arm and hand due to surgical trauma**	1. Able to close hand Able to comb own hair	post-op day 4 ✓	1A. Exercise and positioning per M.D.'s orders B. Get orders if there are none
	2. Altered self-concept due to surgical procedure	2. Verbalize and non-verbal expression: "I can cope with this situation" Do own makeup Have specific plans for prosthesis and grooming Verbalize concern re-close personal relationships	by disch.	2A. Listen. Let patient express feelings and fears B. Check with M.D. regarding Mastectomy Club or Public Health Nurse C. Give specific ideas and in-formation regarding clothes and stores for mastectomy patients D. Allow husband to express concerns. Problem-solve with him. Help him to see his role

*From Mayers M., and El Camino Hospital Nursing Staff, Standard Care Plans, *Vol. I,* 1974. Courtesy of K.P. Medical Systems.[7]

Theory-Based Standard Care Plans

To illustrate how standard care plans can be refined to articulate clearly the theory basis from which they are derived, a revised version of the mastectomy standard-care plan is shown. In this care plan (Fig. 5.2) the problem statements have been rephrased to reflect clearly the theory elements involved. For example, problem 2, based on Selye's theory of stress and the open-systems theory, utilizes the term "psychological stress" from Selye's theory and the term "feedback" from systems theory. Similarly, the expected outcomes are expressed through words and phrases that relate directly to the elements and postulates of the theories. When theories are directly used as guides for practice, nursing orders (interventions) are also influenced.

In the case of problem 2, the nursing orders from the original standard changed because of the nursing theory. The new orders require the nursing interventions to explore alternatives (feedback-systems theory) and require active and reflective listening to foster free self-expression (a postulate required by Selye's psychological stress theory). The reader can similarly analyze the remaining revisions of the care plan to see how theory-related standards directly influence the nurse's cognitive processes, terminology, expected client behavior, and nursing intervention. This direct linkage makes possible evaluation of one nurse's thought processes by a peer. In addition, this ability to trace theory-related thought processes lays the groundwork for developing and verifying nursing theories.

Audit Criteria

Audit criteria are also frequently used as standards for assessment and documentation. These also are generally formulated according to medical and nursing diagnoses. There are various formats for audit criteria and their tabulation. Both directly and indirectly, audit criteria suggest the theories from which they may have been derived. Fig. 5.3 shows one version of audit criteria for the normal newborn.[8]

As was done for the standard care plan, audit criteria can be reviewed and there can be speculation about the underlying theories from which the criteria were developed. In Fig. 5.3, all the admission criteria, 1 through 7, probably refer to the physiological system of man, his normal growth and development. The same is true for the interim and discharge phases. Criterion 12 may also be based on the physiological response to a microbial stressor.

In this figure it can be seen that a conceptual framework, with its theories, can support all the audit criteria written by nurses. However, the theories within the conceptual framework may enlarge the scope of standards because of the many theories required to interpret man. Fig. 5.4 shows a revised version of normal newborn audit criteria, incorporating

Figure 5.2

Theory-Based Standard Care Plan

PROBLEMS	EXPECTED OUTCOMES	DEADLINES	NURSING ORDERS
Pre-Op			
1. Standard†	1. Standard		1. Standard
2. Psychological stress due to unavailable feedback regarding prognosis. (Based on Selye's theory of stress and open-systems theory requiring a feedback loop.)	2. Verbalizes possible prognostic alternatives. Expresses own feelings freely. (Both behaviors represent feedback which is a requirement of both theories.)	Pre-op or when confirmed path report available.	2A. Explore with client the various alternatives that are likely. B. Active and reflective listening to foster free self-expression.
Early Post-Op			
1. Shock, denial, or anger due to loss of body part. (Based on Kubler-Ross's stages of grief, 1 and 2.)	2. Exhibits "bargaining" behavior. (This outcome represents passage into the third stage of grief.)	√ q̄ shift.	1A. Allow acting-out behavior, but do not reinforce denial. B. Allow some dependency. C. Expect expressions of anger, do not personalize them.
2. Potential hypostatic pneumonia due to compensatory splinting. (Based on physiological theories of pain and mobility.)	2. Has clear lung sounds. (This outcome represents adequate lung expansion-mobility.)	√ q̄ shift.	2A. Check lung sounds q̄ 2h according to physical exam guide. B. Check V.S. q̄ 4h. C. Turn, cough and deep-breathe q̄ 2h for first 24 hrs then q̄ 4h.

Nursing Diagnosis	Outcomes	Time	Actions
			D. Administer pain med prior to turn, cough and deep breathe. E. Ambulate frequently. F. Check dressings for constriction.
Late Post-Op 1. Potential short- and long-term limited mobility of affected hand and arm due to surgical trauma. (Based on physiological theory of mobility and movement.)	1. Uses affected hand and arm for activities of daily living. Has minimal or no edema of hand and arm. (Outcomes relative to joint movement and transport systems.)	After 24 hrs By discharge √ daily A.M. & P.M.	1A. Avoid abduction for first week. Begin flexion and extension of wrist and elbow $\bar{q}$ h starting during first 24 hrs. B. Require use of affected arm for ADL.
2. Potential thwarting of female sexuality and goal fulfillment due to altered self-perception. (Based on Day's theory of perception and Sarbin's theory of reciprocal interaction.)	2. Verbalizes choices available to achieve satisfaction and goal-fulfillment in female role. Verbalizes positive interactions with significant others. Outcomes represent behaviors reflecting self-perception and reciprocal interactions.)	By discharge	2A. Encourage free expression of meanings and values relative to sexuality. B. Explore personal goals to achieve satisfaction. C. Discuss theory of reciprocal interaction as it affects client and how client can control.

†*This refers to a set of nursing diagnoses and actions that would be typical for any pre-operative patient based on physiological, psychological, and cognitive/intellectual systems of man. Not illustrated here.*

new criteria required by theories embodied within the conceptual framework.[9]

Assessment Guides

Just as audit criteria and standard care plans are used as guides for assessment and documentation, so are nursing histories. Over the years, nursing histories have taken many different forms. Some have been very brief and related to a few crucial observations and a few basic questions. Others represent a general body-systems review, while still others are much longer and more detailed, and incorporate many questions and observations relating to a more holistic approach to man. In 1971, Orem published a conceptual model for patient care which focused on man's needs for self-care.[10] This model requires nursing to assist man as his own health-care agent. Related to this function, the information or data-gathering guide used by the nurse

> ...will include the description of (1) the degree of the patient's illness, its causes, and whether it is acute or chronic; (2) obvious injuries or defects; (3) the patient's present behavior patterns (what he does or does not do); (4) the effects of disease or disordered function being experienced by the patient (including pain, alterations of body temperature, alterations of respiratory and circulatory functioning, gastrointestinal functioning, genitourinary functioning, nervous and musculo-skeletal functioning, alterations of the skin and its appendages, and bleeding and anemia);[11] and (5) possible or known effects of the patient's present health state on his future capacity for effective living.[10]

Orem's assessment guide is specifically designed to relate to the theories which support the self-care philosophy; thus her assessment guide is theory-related.

Another example of a direct theory-related assessment guide is that developed by Betty Neuman in her "Health Care Systems Model: A Total Approach To Patient Problems."[12] Her total-person approach requires specific assessment of each element in her concept of a person. Each question or observation relates directly to one or more element of her model. Fig. 5.5 shows this model and the related assessment guide.[12] Many detailed assessment guidelines are set forth in a discussion of the total model.

Most existing assessment guides are not this directly theory-related. One can, however, speculate some relationship to theories in many of them. An example of one that is not specifically theory-related is Part I of a nursing history suggested by Murray[13] and illustrated in Fig. 5.6. The first section of Murray's nursing history suggests 12 questions, each designed to gain information about the patient's perceptions and expectations of his illness and hospitalization. One can infer that questions 1 through 6 are derived from ethnocentric theory. Questions 7, 8, 9, and 10 hint at Sullivan's

Figure 5.3
Audit Criteria for Normal Newborn**[8]

DIAGNOSTIC CATEGORY: Normal Newborn

Standards/Criteria	Percent Desired Compliance	Predictable Exceptions	Instructions to Auditor
Admission: (First 15 minutes)			
1. APGAR Score	100	None	Nurses' admission notes or flow sheet
2. Reflexes: rooting, pupillary, palmar grasp, moro, neck rigidity.	100	None	Nurses' admission notes or flow sheet
3. Temperature, rectal.	100	None	Nurses' admission notes or flow sheet
4. Meconium; absence or presence.	100	None	Nurses' admission notes or flow sheet
5. Status of cord: length and absence or presence of bleeding.	100	None	Nurses' admission notes or flow sheet
6. Status of fontanels: size in cm. and tension.	100	None	Nurses' admission notes or flow sheet
7. Amount of oral mucous: none, moderate, or excessive.	100	None	Nurses' admission notes or flow sheet
Interim: (After first 15 minutes through day 2)			
8. Body temperature above 97 F by 8 hr post-delivery.	100	None	Flow sheet
9. Description of respiration rate and rhythm q̄ 8 hr.	100	None	Flow sheet

Figure 5.3 *(cont.)*

Audit Criteria for Normal Newborn**[8]

DIAGNOSTIC CATEGORY: NORMAL NEWBORN

STANDARDS/CRITERIA	PERCENT DESIRED COMPLIANCES	PREDICTABLE EXCEPTIONS	INSTRUCTIONS TO AUDITOR
10. Response to feeding after feeding at least q̄ 6 hr.	100	None	Flow sheet
Discharge: (Day of discharge)			
11. Taking and retaining prescribed fluids well.	100	None	Nurses' notes or flow sheet
12. Cord clean and intact.	100	None	Nurses' notes or flow sheet
13. Body weight approximates birth weight (acceptable variance per nursery protocol).	100	None	Nurses' notes or flow sheet

**Adapted from Mayers, Norby and Watson: Quality Assurance for Patient Care, Nursing Perspectives, 1977, p 253. Courtesy of Appleton-Century-Crofts, publisher.

Figure 5.4
Theory-Based Audit Criteria‡

DIAGNOSTIC CATEGORY: NORMAL NEWBORN
      ADMISSION: (FIRST 15 MINUTES)

1. APGAR Score — at 1″ and 5″
2. Quality of cry — feeble, high-pitched
3. Temperature — unusually high or low
4. Bonding behaviors of baby:
   - Looks at mother's face
   - Eyes follow hand movement
   - Smiles at mother
   - Turns head toward mother's voice
   - Cuddles in toward mother's heart sounds
5. Bonding behavior of mother:
   - Physical holding, rhythmic movement
   - Gazing and eye contact
   - Caressing starting with fingertips, then palms
   - Cuddles to breast
   - Entertains baby with high-pitched voice

    (Behaviors 4 and 5 are new criteria added from the interactive/ affiliative system of man)

6. Reflexes: rooting, pupillary, palmar grasp, moro and neck rigidity.
7. Meconium, absence or presence.
8. Status of cord, length and absence or presence of bleeding.
9. Status of fontanels, size in cm. and tension.
10. Amount of oral mucous: none, moderate, or excessive.

    (Criteria 6 through 10 are based on the physiological system of man, systems theory)

INTERIM (FROM FIRST 15 MINUTES THROUGH DAY 2)

11. Body temperature above 97° F by 8 hours post-delivery.
12. Description of respiration, rate and rhythm q8h.
13. Response to feeding at least q6h.

    (Criteria 11 through 13 are based on a body systems review of man)

14. Continued bonding behaviors of mother and infant, see criteria 4 and 5.

DISCHARGE (DAY OF DISCHARGE)

15. Taking and retaining prescribed fluids well.

    (Based on theories of growth and development, and systems.)

16. Cord clean and intact.

    (Based on Selye's theory of stress and the body's response to a microbial stressor.)

> **Figure 5.4** *(cont.)*
> Theory-Based Audit Criteria‡
>
> DIAGNOSTIC CATEGORY: NORMAL NEWBORN
>   ADMISSION: (FIRST 15 MINUTES)
>
> 17. Body weight approximate birth weight.
>   (Based on physiological systems theory, and growth and development.)
> 18. Mother's behavior characterizes caring: urge to have baby with her, touching, holding, talking to, nursing/feeding, responding to cry, centering attention on baby.
>   (Based on Erickson's theory of psychological development, phase one, trust versus mistrust.)
>
> ‡*From Mayers, Norby, and Watson8*

interpersonal theory. And questions 11 and 12 can be construed to relate to role theory. This assessment guide is general in nature. Many assessment guides are specifically developed to meet the needs of a given situation or a particular client population. Appendix C shows several examples of this.

Analysis

From the previously cited examples, it is suggested that the nurse may be able to revise her existing care plans, audit criteria, and assessment guides in order to be more directly theory-related. If she revises her care plans according to a theory base, the same theory elements will obviously apply to other assessment and documentation tools. Thus, if it is not realistic or feasible to construct an entire conceptual framework and to begin everything from scratch, it is possible to work inductively, gradually filling in theory-by-theory those concepts that ultimately become the guide for nursing practice—the conceptual framework.

IMPLICATION FOR POLICIES

Policies also guide nursing practice and should ideally be derived from the conceptual framework. A policy is a tool for making operational the conceptual framework, and regulating practice and performance. More specifically, a policy is a written rule formulated to achieve a defined purpose. It is designed to guide behavior and decisions under specific circumstances. Since every agency, and the units within an agency, must have policies, and since policies are influential, they provide a strong potential for implementing theory-based practice.

Man, The Client

Policies on a nursing unit will change when a new theory is formally adopted or recognized. The theory of mother-infant bonding[9] has changed many policies regulating the care of the newborn and the mother. Before this theory was recognized, a delivery room and nursery might have policies that would require immediately placing a baby in a heated crib and whisking him away to the nursery. Upon entry to the nursery, the baby would be stripped, washed, inspected, and placed in a little plastic bin. Meanwhile, the mother was stranded in the recovery room, wondering what happened to her baby but hesitant to ask. In all probability she would see and hold him at the next scheduled feeding period, which could be from two to six hours later. All these events would have occurred as a direct result of policies governing practice in the delivery room, nursery, and recovery room. The policies were intended to insure safe care. For instance the baby was whisked away to make sure the experts in the nursery could properly evaluate his condition. The mother was sent to the recovery room to make sure her post-delivery status was properly monitored. The feeding schedule was determined in accordance with the constraints of the setting—time, logistics, staff—and perhaps an epidemiologic rationale. The father has not been mentioned at all in this situation. Quite typically, he is sitting downstairs by himself, wondering what is going on. By policy, he is barred from contact with mother and infant.

Policies which reflect bonding theory create a different scenario. A delivery room looks different—softer, more homelike, less distracting. The father may be present. The baby is immediately placed in the mother's arms or on her chest, allowing for cradling, gazing, and talking. The staff behaves differently. They avoid distracting the family during these crucial moments of bonding. The baby can accompany the mother to the recovery room, which has beds large enough to accommodate both. One can go further to delineate changes in policy based on bonding and family theory. The mother, father, and infant are treated as an active family throughout the course of hospitalization.

On a medical unit, the impact on policy and practice of adoption of the Kubler-Ross theory of grief and dying[14] can be imagined. For instance the client's values and concerns then take precedence over typical unit routines. The family may assume a much more active role in care. And the nurse may truly have to function as an advocate to discover the client's choice of those he wants to spend his final time with. Policies consistent with the theory allow for maximum flexibility and freedom of client mobility within and outside the agency, provision for a homelike or comforting environment, and psychological support systems for client, family, and staff. One obvious outcome of this kind of theory is the development of hospice and home-care programs for the terminally ill.

Convalescent care policies change when theories of biological rhythms

Figure 5.5

Betty Neuman's Health-Care Systems Model: A Total Approach to Patient Problems.*[12]

'PHYSIOLOGICAL, PSYCHOLOGICAL, SOCIOCULTURAL, AND DEVELOPMENTAL FACTORS OCCUR AND ARE CONSIDERED SIMULTANEOUSLY

BASIC STRUCTURE
BASIC FACTORS COMMON TO ALL ORGANISMS. I.E.,
• NORMAL TEMPERATURE RANGE
• GENETIC STRUCTURE
• RESPONSE PATTERN
• ORGAN STRENGTH
• WEAKNESS
• EGO STRUCTURE
• KNOWNS OR COMMONALITIES

STRESSORS
• MORE THAN ONE STRESSOR CAN OCCUR SIMULTANEOUSLY'
• SAME STRESSOR CAN VARY AS TO IMPACT OR REACTION
• NORMAL DEFENSE LINE VARIES WITH AGE AND DEVELOPMENT

STRESSOR

STRESSOR

STRESSOR

FLEXIBLE LINE OF DEFENSE

NORMAL LINE OF DEFENSE

LINES OF 'RESISTANCE

BASIC STRUCTURE ENERGY RESOURCES

DEGREE OF REACTION

RECONSTITUTION

RECONSTITUTION
• COULD BEGIN AT ANY DEGREE OR LEVEL OF REACTION
• RANGE OF POSSIBILITY MAY EXTEND BEYOND NORMAL LINE OF DEFENSE

INTRA
INTER
EXTRA
PERSONAL FACTORS

STRESSORS
• IDENTIFIED
• CLASSIFIED AS TO KNOWNS OR POSSIBILITIES. I.E.,
• LOSS
• PAIN
• SENSORY DEPRIVATION
• CULTURAL CHANGE

INTRA
INTER
EXTRA
PERSONAL FACTORS

REACTION

REACTION
• INDIVIDUAL INTERVENING VARIABLES. I.E.,
• BASIC STRUCTURE IDIOSYNCRASIES
• NATURAL AND LEARNED RESISTANCE
• TIME OF ENCOUNTER WITH STRESSOR

INTRA
INTER
EXTRA
PERSONAL FACTORS

INTERVENTIONS
• CAN OCCUR BEFORE OR AFTER RESISTANCE LINES ARE PENETRATED IN BOTH REACTION AND RECONSTITUTION PHASES
• INTERVENTIONS ARE BASED ON:
• DEGREE OF REACTION
• RESOURCES
• GOALS
• ANTICIPATED OUTCOME

PRIMARY PREVENTION
• REDUCE POSSIBILITY OF ENCOUNTER WITH STRESSORS
• STRENGTHEN FLEXIBLE LINE OF DEFENSE

SECONDARY PREVENTION
• EARLY CASE-FINDING AND
• TREATMENT OF SYMPTOMS

TERTIARY PREVENTION
• READAPTATION
• REEDUCATION TO PREVENT FUTURE OCCURRENCES
• MAINTENANCE OF STABILITY

Primary Prevention	Secondary Prevention	Tertiary Prevention
Stressors* Mainly covert. Reaction Hypothetical. Assessment Based on patient assessment, experience, and theory. Data should include: 1. Risks or possible hazards to the patient based on patient/nurse perception. 2. Meaning of the experience to the patient. 3. Life-style factors. 4. Coping patterns (past-present-possible). 5. Individual differences. 6. Other. Interventions Strengthen resistance to the hazard by: 1. Education. 2. Desensitization. 3. Avoidance of hazard. 4. Strengthening of individual resistance factors.	Stressors† Mainly overt or known. Reaction Identified by symptomatology or known factors. Assessment Determine nature and degree of reaction. Determine internal/external resources available to resist the reaction. Rationale for goals — with collaborative goal-setting with the patient when possible. Interventions Based on the following: 1. Ranking of priority of needs related to symptoms. 2. Patient strengths and weaknesses as related to the "4" variables.† 3. Shift of priorities needed as the patient responds to treatment or as the nature of stressors change. (Primary prevention needs may occur simultaneously with treatment or secondary prevention.) 4. Need to deal with maladaptive processes. 5. Optimum use of internal/external resources, i.e. conservation of energy, noise reduction, financial aid.	Stressors† Mainly overt or residual — covert factors a possibility. Reaction Hypothetical or known — residual symptoms or factors. Assessment Degree of stability following treatment; possible further reconstitution level assessed. Possible regression factors. Interventions May include: 1. Motivation. 2. Reeducation. 3. Behavior modification. 4. Reality orientation. 5. Progressive goal-setting. 6. Optimal use of appropriate available resources. 7. Maintenance of a reasonable adaptive level of functioning.

*From Riehl and Roy: Conceptual Models for Nursing Practice, 1974, pp 100, 106. Courtesy of Appleton-Century-Crofts, publishers.
†Assessment should include information concerning the relationship of the four variables: physiologic, psychologic, sociocultural, and developmental.

Figure 5.6
Nursing History, Indirectly Theory-Related**[13]

Nursing History

Date: *February 18, 1975*
Name: *Meg Rogers*
Hospital Number: *123-34-0155*
Address (city or county): *Sunnyside*
Age: *32*   Sex: M   F *X*
Occupation: *Teacher's Aide*
Religion: *Methodist*
Race/National Origin: *American Negro*
Medical Diagnosis: *Toxoplasmosis, Detached Retina, rt. eye*
Information obtained from Patient: *X*
Other: *X*
Relationship: *husband*
History needs to be rechecked at later date: *Check postsurgical*

I. Patient Perceptions and Expectations Related to Illness/Hospitalization

1. Why did you come to the hospital? (or go to the doctor?)
   Spots in front of right eye and diminished vision.

2. What do you think caused you to get sick?
   Toxoplasmosis, which preceded detached retina (patient thinks it was caused by eating raw or rare meat or having a cat).

3. Has being sick made any difference in your usual way of life? If so, how?
   The medication I have been taking has made me tired. I am now more careful about the way I use my eyes and try to read for shorter periods of time.

4. What do you expect is going to happen to you in the hospital?
   I will be operated upon for reattachment of retina, and I will remain in hospital for 4 days' recupteration.

5. What is it like for you being in the hospital?
   It's neither good nor bad. I want to get this operation over with quickly and have the problem taken care of so that I can go back to a normal life. The doctors and nurses are professional and answer questions, but brusquely. The surroundings are comfortable.

6. How long do you expect to be in the hospital?
   3-4 days

7. With whom do you live?
   Husband and 2 children (ages 3 and 7)

Figure 5.6 *(cont.)*
Nursing History, Indirectly Theory-Related**[13]

8. Who is the most important person(s) to you?
   Husband and children

9. What effect has your coming to the hospital had on your family? (or closest person?)
   The normal family routine has been upset in many ways. Friends, relatives, and babysitters are all pitching in to help out during hospitalization by cooking meals, getting children off to school, helping husband with house chores. However, house seems to be in a "holding pattern" until my return.

10. Are any of your family (or close persons) able to visit you in the hospital?
    Yes, husband and friends will visit. Children will not. Husband can only come on weekend because of working hours.

11. What do you enjoy doing for recreation? (to pass the time?)
    Reading, writing, sewing, sports, card-playing.

12. How do you expect to get along after you leave the hospital?
    I think it will be difficult because of the demands on my time and services (housework, cooking, taking care of children, dependency on car to get around and to chauffeur kids). I realize it will be difficult to do all these things as before, and I guess I will have to get some help, but I don't know where.

**From Murray: Fundamentals of Nursing,[13] *1976, p 82. Courtesy of Prentice-Hall Publishing Co., Inc. Revised in accordance with directions of Prentice-Hall, Inc., in signed permission.*

---

are recognized and adopted. No longer do policies require that all clients be tucked in by 9:00 P.M. to sleep soundly until 6:00 A.M., at which time everyone wakens to eat breakfast. Instead, flexibility relative to the individual's biological rhythms and normal life style dictate schedules and activities.

The previous examples illustrate the relationship among theories, policies, and practice. Obviously three examples which vividly illustrate the point have been chosen. The ramifications and generalizations are infinite. Not only does the conceptual framework provide theories which interpret man the client; they also interpret man the care-provider within a specified setting. Therefore, both the client and the care-provider are regulated by the conceptual framework.

Man, the Care-Provider

With or without a conceptual framework, decisions must be made regarding the care-provider (learner). It must be decided who is responsible for what, who does what, when something is to be done, and how it is to be done. Levels of competency and expectation must in some way be determined. For example, how should clients be assessed, who should assess them, what information should be gathered, when should assessment occur, and finally, what should be done with the information? Policies provide the answers. They are more easily developed, written, implemented, and monitored when there is a theoretical framework as a basis. This basis explains the purpose and rationale for governing decisions relative to levels of competency and expectations.

In both the educational and service settings there are performers and learners with different degrees of knowledge. They must be held accountable for different levels of competency. In the service setting, this may be a registered nurse progressing from a probationary level to staff nurse 2 or 3. Levels of competency may also be defined among classifications of workers—attendant, L.V.N., R.N., clinical specialist—with uncommon sequences of expectations and responsibility. In the educational setting, student learning experiences, performance objectives, and competency expectations are also sequential in levels relative to the knowledge necessary to perform at a given point. For example, the student may be held accountable for "application" of five theories relative to man at the end of the first clinical semester and "synthesis" and "evaluation" of 18 theories relative to man and the environment upon completion of a total learning program.

Levels of competency can be derived from the learning theories which explain man within the nurse's conceptual framework. She may note that student expectations progress from application to synthesis and evaluation. Basically, these terms are theory elements from Bloom's taxonomy of cognitive development.[15] He theorizes that learning progresses sequentially from recalling facts (knowledge), to explaining (comprehension), to using facts in new situations (application), to gathering multiple facts and determining alternative causes of action (analysis and synthesis), and finally to judging (evaluation). This taxonomy is almost universally used in educational settings to define levels of cognitive competency relative to theoretical formulations. Many nursing-service settings use the same taxonomy to define performance expectations and job descriptions.

Assessment, as interpreted here, results in a nursing diagnosis, which is defined as a judgment or defensible conclusion. This definition clearly requires competency at the highest cognitive level, that of evaluation. Therefore, the job description for a registered nurse may clearly specify this performance expectation relative to assessment and documentation. By contrast, it can be expected that other care-providers with different educational preparation will demonstrate other levels of cognitive competence relative to assessment and documentation. With this theoretical rationale, it becomes much easier to specify which level of performer assesses and documents which aspects of client care. These expectations are set forth in policies related to admission (nursing histories), care-planning, and charting—to mention a few.

Levels of competency are considered here only in relation to cognitive expectations of assessment and documentation. In reality, job descriptions will specify affective and psychomotor competencies relative to assessment and documentation and many other elements of practice, each reflecting some component of the conceptual framework.

Man, a Member of the Organization

The overall organization also has policies that determine how it interacts with its employees, how it makes decisions, and how authority and accountability are established. These policies can represent arbitrary decisions or can be consistent with a conceptual framework. Again, the construct, concepts, and theories guide policy formulation. If an organization embraces the theory that man is an active, positive, satisfaction-seeking being with variable amounts of energy[16], its policies are different from those of an organization that views man as a passive, self-seeking worker. Acting on the first theory, an organization may prescribe for itself personnel policies that reward employees for achievement rather than for longevity. A variety of rewards can be used: money; recognition; freedom for creativity; scheduling; flexibility for research, writing, planning, and so forth. Participative evaluations take the place of superior-to-subordinate reviews. Management objectives are negotiated rather than handed down. Organization decisions are made through participative or consensus methods, rather than unilaterally by the "person at the top." This theory may also lead an organization to remove some of the layers of its hierarchy, delegating authority to the most knowledgeable people wherever they may be within the organizational structure. Conversely, in an organization which adopts the theory of man as a passive, self-seeking worker, hierarchal authority relationships may be more valid. Only one theory has been used to illustrate a point, but many others can be relevant to the policies an organization develops to guide its own actions.

Organizational policy is not unique to formal administrative positions. The nurse at the bedside has a component of administration in her daily activities, as does the team leader, head nurse, primary-care nurse, and the director of nursing. A nurse who operates under the theory of man as an active, positive being includes her clients in decisions that involve them, delegates some authority to the clients themselves, and participates in joint decision-making.

Thus, the conceptual framework serves to guide the nurse at any level of practice—the practitioner with her clients, the nurse-manager with her staff, the faculty member with her students, and the nurse administrator with her organization. The same constructs, concepts, and theories provide the basis for each level of competency and for performance expectations whatever the personnel classification. Each employee (learner) within a given setting knows what is expected of him relative to the predictable characteristics of each construct and concept. In return, the employee (learner) knows what to expect of the organization and what his role is within the structure. This then provides the foundation for evaluation and accountability at all levels of nursing practice.

IMPLICATIONS FOR EVALUATION

"The purpose of evaluation is always that of determining the worth or value of something. In the context of...nursing...the purpose is to determine that worthwhile patient effects or 'outcomes' are occurring."[8] Evaluation occurs through initial, ongoing, and final assessment. Evaluation information is the feedback data used to make decisions and judgments affecting subsequent interventions. Measurement is implied whenever evaluation occurs. To measure something, yardsticks, such as standards, must be defined.

It will be remembered that standards are derived from criteria (theory elements) and they establish a value. Values are established in one of three ways: group norms; experts' opinions; or individual expectations. The literature tends to refer to group norms as norm-referenced evaluation, and to expert and individual opinions as criterion-referenced.[17] Whenever the nurse evaluates an individual's performance or outcome against specific behavioral objectives, she is using criterion-referenced evaluation. Whenever she evaluates an individual's status against mathematically determined group values, she is using norm-referenced evaluation. Both are applicable in nursing.

Client Evaluation

Client evaluation occurs at various times and in several ways. For example, upon admission to a service a client is evaluated to establish "baseline" status. Many of the assessment guides in this text provide examples of initial evaluation. Periodic evaluation occurs subsequently, sometimes hour-by-hour, or day-by-day, or at less frequent intervals. Care plans with their expected outcomes and deadlines (objectives) exemplify this periodic evaluation process. Actual patient status, compared with desired status or expected outcomes, indicates a client's changing or improving level of health. This documented evidence of health status is used for both concurrent and retrospective evaluation.

Concurrent evaluation refers to "those processes that are designed to evaluate care that is still in progress."[8] Concurrent evaluation can be done for an individual client, or collectively for a group of clients. Measurement methodologies can include open chart audits, client and staff interviews, care-plan audits, bedside audits, or standardized tests.

Final client outcomes, individual or collective, can be evaluated retrospectively when an episode of care is completed. Methodologies may include closed chart reviews, post-care patient interviews, and staff conferences, or questionnaires. Measurement tools for both retrospective and concurrent evaluation may be either norm-referenced or criterion-referenced.

The entire previous discussion refers to periodic, longitudinal evaluation over a span of time. Within each time span, levels of competency are evaluated. For example, if a client has a problem in the cognitive/intellectual domain, his changing status can be measured periodically through a hierarchy, such as in Bloom's *Taxonomy*.[15] Early in his learning period, he may be evaluated for having achieved comprehension, later for application and analysis, and finally for synthesis and evaluation. As illustration of psychomotor development,[17,18] or use of manual skills, the nurse can consider a new mother learning to give her newborn a bath. Any client education must evaluate an individual's skills relative to some theory-related level of competency. Theory-based evaluation, then, can ultimately lead nurses to identify progressive levels of competency for all the systems of man.

Learner and Care-Provider Evaluation

Learner evaluation also occurs at various times and in different ways. Upon admission to a nursing-education program, students are evaluated to determine their basic competence. Admission standards are the guidelines for these judgments. Periodic evaluation occurs subsequently at various levels in the curriculum. A faculty may decide that all students should exhibit certain competency levels upon completion of prerequisites to the nursing major, and can define these competencies as a level. Subsequent phases may be designated as levels 2, 3, and 4. Each level builds upon preceding levels. More frequent evaluation occurs during and after each course within each level. Individual student performance is compared with standards, referred to as course and level behaviors. If the faculty evaluates students according to behavioral objectives, they are involved in criterion-referenced evaluation. Norm-referenced evaluation may also be used when an adequate sample of predictable competencies can be extrapolated. Examples of well-known norm-referenced evaluation tools are the national league for nursing achievement examination and college entrance examinations.

Within each time frame, course, or level, competence is evaluated according to the theory introduced at that point. Theories are selectively placed in the curriculum according to the faculties' beliefs about the learner, the educational setting, and the basis of knowledge necessary for practice. As with the client, levels of cognitive, affective, and psychomotor development, can be measured through such a hierarchy as revealed in Bloom's *Taxonomy*.[15,18,19] Competence expectations are also derived from the faculties' definition of learning as made operational in their conceptual framework. If, for instance, a group believes learning should progress from "simple to complex," content, learning experiences and evaluation are developed and introduced accordingly. As an example, the beginning student may be expected to include simple physical assessment skills in the examination of one client in a simulated setting, whereas a fourth-level student may be expected to use more physical assessment skills as part of the complete assessment of each client in a real intensive-care setting.

Methods of student evaluation take many forms. Common examples are teacher-made tests, standardized achievement tests, student-teacher conferences, observation of performance, student logs and diaries, anecdotal notes, self-evaluation or employer-employee questionnaires. These methods may reflect either criterion-referenced or norm-referenced evaluation, or both.

Evaluation of competency for practitioners is similar to that for the client and student in terms of time and level.[20] In the service setting, a practitioner is evaluated in relation to beginning employment standards, in order to identify baseline competency. Periodic evaluation occurs at regular intervals throughout an entire episode of employment. Early evaluation occurs during or by the end of a probationary period, which may be considered analogous to a beginning level. The conceptual framework of a nursing service, its beliefs and theories about man as a care-provider and man as a client, and the agency and its environment, all guide the evaluation process.

Organization Evaluation

To remain in harmony with her conceptual framework, the nurse also needs to evaluate her organization. Do actual personnel practices comply with the policies derived from the theories? Are decision-making processes consistent with the theories articulated in the conceptual framework? Are performance objectives being met? Is delegated authority left inviolate? Measurement methods which can be used to evaluate and find answers to these questions include staff and faculty questionnaires; conferences; evaluation of staff, faculty, and learner performances; measurement of client outcomes; and attitudinal studies. It may be possible to find some standardized, norm-referenced, tests that relate closely enough to one's theory to be justifiably used as a measurement tool. In the absence of appropriate standardized tests, experts can compose measurement tools that are theory-related and that can be used to evaluate the organization's actions.

IMPLICATIONS FOR THE FUTURE

Nursing, as a profession, has not conducted enough research or gathered enough data to establish norms which enable prediction of client and nurse behavior. This deficiency in the body of knowledge provides a direction for the future.

Yet, every day, millions of nurses are making predictions about their clients and about their own nursing interventions. How does a nurse know that her client should be ambulatory 12 hours postoperatively? How does she know that if she turns someone every two hours, she will substantially reduce the potential for an embolism? How does she know that if she spends 20 minutes every shift letting a person express his feelings, he will experience less anxiety? How does she know that it is valuable to provide the post-coronary client with a specific teaching plan while he is still hospitalized? How does she know that a client's family will exhibit grief when told of the client's impending death?

As the questions are posed, nurses say: "Of course we can explain and predict many of these things." We can reiterate the physiological theories and the research evidence that explains much physiological behavior. Because of these theories we are confident as we assess, intervene, and evaluate. Our confidence diminishes somewhat when we are confronted with a need to predict outcomes of an emotional, interactional, psychological, intellectual, and perceptive nature. And yet much of our time, energy, concern, and commitment lies in these areas. We also see that our clients look to us for support, reassurance, security, and some predictability when they are frightened, unable to cope, unable to understand what is happening, or unable to think and plan.

The attempt here has been to formulate norms to use as guides for assessing all the systems of man. It is relatively easy to find established norms in books and references for the physiological system. However, as the literature and theories relating to the other systems of man are studied, few, if any, numerical norms are found to enable definition of standards for assessment and evaluation. These other systems of man cry out for investigation and analysis from the nursing perspective. Nurses at the bedside have a built-in opportunity to study man's responses to his environment—to treatment, culture, health, physical effects, and so forth.

What is suggested is that nurses in many situations are always observing, studying, and generalizing. This is, of course, informal research, the building of a personal body of knowledge. Formalizing this process leads to development of a professional body of knowledge. King reveals the right method for compilation by a profession of a body of knowledge.

Theory, models, and methods relevant for nursing will be developed and used by nurses to conduct research that will predict the behavior of individuals in complex health-care systems. Tomorrow's nurses will be expected to solve problems in the complex systems being established today. They will be expected to predict, and thus, to prevent problems from occurring as well as to plan for adaptation for emergencies of life. Nurses will describe the bio-psycho-social aspects of human behavior and explain the interdependence of these factors. Theories for nursing will become the common denominator for practice, teaching, and research.[21]

The authors here believe that theory-building and theory-testing offer nursing an answer to its dilemma. Theoretical formulations incorporated into a conceptual framework provide a common language enabling nurses to learn from each other, and, perhaps more important, to articulate, explain, and justify their role within society. A common language opens the doors to definition of the boundaries of nursing, to collaboration with others, and to more accurate assessment, prediction, evaluation, and advancement of nursing practice.

REFERENCES

1. Chater S: A conceptual framework for curriculum development. *Nurs Outlook* 23:7:428-433, July 1975.
2. Chater S: A conceptual framework as a basis for decisions about teaching strategies. Paper presented at COGEN (Cooperative Graduate Education in Nursing) San Francisco, Calif, 1973, p 6.
3. Argyris C, Schon D: *Theory In Practice: Increasing Professional Effectiveness.* San Francisco, Calif, Jossey-Bass Publishers, 1974, pp 3-19.
4. Davidson S: *Nursing Care Evaluation, Concurrent and Retrospective Review Criteria.* St Louis, CV Mosby Co, 1977, p VIII.
5. Gebbe K, Lavin M: *Classification of Nursing Diagnoses.* St Louis, CV Mosby Co, 1975.
6. Gebbe K: *Summary of Second National Conference, Classification of Nursing Diagnosis.* St Louis, National Group for Classification of Nursing Diagnoses, 1976.
7. Mayers, M, El Camino Hospital Nursing Staff: *Standard Care Plans,* Vol 1, Stockton, Calif, K/P Co Medical Systems, 1974, p 6.
8. Mayers M, Norby R, Watson A: *Quality Assurance For Patient Care: Nursing Perspectives.* New York, Appleton-Century-Crofts, 1977, pp 87, 253.
9. Klaus M, Kennell J: *Maternal-Infant Bonding.* St Louis, CV Mosby Co, 1976, pp 68-80.
10. Orem D: *Nursing Concepts of Practice.* New York, McGraw-Hill Book Co, 1971, pp 159-160.
11. Harrison T, et al: *Principles of Internal Medicine.* 5th ed, New York, McGraw-Hill Book Co, 1966.
12. Neuman B: The Betty Neuman health care systems model: A total person approach to patient problems. In Reihl J, Roy C: *Conceptual Models for Nursing Practice.* New York, Appleton-Century-Crofts, 1974, pp 99-112.
13. Murray M: *Fundamental of Nursing.* Englewood Cliffs, NJ, Prentice-Hall Inc, 1976, p 82.
14. Kubler-Ross E: *On Death and Dying.* New York, The Macmillan Co, 1969.
15. Bloom B, et al: *Taxonomy of Educational Objectives, Handbook I: Cognitive Domain.* New York, David McKay Co, Inc, 1956.
16. McGregor D: *The Human Side of Enterprise.* New York, McGraw-Hill, 1960.

17. Guinee K: *Teaching and Learning in Nursing.* New York, Macmillan Publishing Company, Inc, 1978, pp 36, 47-50.
18. Tuckman B: A four-domain taxonomy for classifying educational tasks and objectives. *Educ Technology* 12:12:36-38, December 1972.
19. Krathwohl D: *Taxonomy of Educational Objectives, Handbook II: Affective Domain.* New York, David McKay Co, Inc, 1964.
20. Tescher B, Colavecchio R: Definition of a standard for clinical nursing practice. *JONA* 7:3:32, March 1977.
21. King I: Toward the future in nursing research. In Batey M (ed): *Communicating Nursing Research, The Research Critique.* Boulder, Colo, Western Interstate Commission for Higher Education, 1968, p 159.

BIBLIOGRAPHY

Arndt C, Huckabay L: *Nursing Administration: Theory for Practice With a Systems Approach.* St Louis, CV Mosby Co, 1975.

Bayer M, Brandner P: Nurse-patient peer practice. *Am J Nurs* 77:1:86-90, January 1977.

Benoliel J: The interaction between theory and research. *Nurs Outlook* 25:2:108-113, February 1977.

Block D: Criteria, standards, norms—crucial terms in quality assurance. *J Nurs Adm* 7:7:20-29, September 1977.

Bronowski J: Science as foresight. In Neuman J (ed): *What is Science?* New York, Simon and Schuster, 1955.

Davidson G: Coordination of nursing service and nursing education. In *Collaboration for Quality Health Care: Education of Beginning Practitioners of Nursing and Utilization of Graduates.* New York, National League for Nursing, 1977, pp 25-27.

Dickerson T: Roles and responsibilities for nursing service. In *Collaboration for Quality Health Care: Education of Beginning Practitioners of Nursing and Utilization of Graduates.* New York, National League for Nursing, 1977, pp 29-36.

Ethridge P, Packard R: An innovative approach to measurement of quality through utilization of nursing care plans. *J Nurs Adm* 6:1:76:25, January 1976.

Fine R: Nursing roles and responsibilities in a democratic environment. In *Collaboration for Quality Health Care: Education of Beginning Practitioners of Nursing and Utilization of Graduates.* New York, National League for Nursing, 1977, pp 55-60.

Folta J: Obfuscation of clarification: A reaction to Walker's concept of nursing theory. *Nurs Res* 20:496, November-December 1976.

Hamrick A, Greshan M, Eccard M: Staff evaluation of clinical leaders. *J Nurs Adm* 8:1:18-26, January 1978.

Hodgman E: Conceptual framework to guide nursing curriculum. *Nurs Forum* 12:2:110, 1973.

Johnson D: Development of theory: A requisite for nursing as a primary health profession. *Nurs Res* 23:5:372-377, September-October 1974.

Ketefian S: A paradigm for faculty evaluation. *Nurs Outlook* 25:11:718-720, November 1977.

Klaus M, et al: Material attachment: Importance of the first postpartum days. *N Engl J Med* 281:461, 1962.

Klein J: Theory development in nursing. In Chaska N (ed): *The Nursing Profession: Views Through the Mist.* New York, McGraw-Hill Book Co, 1978, pp 223-231.

Laros J: Deriving outcome criteria from a conceptual model. *Nurs Outlook* 25:5:333-336, May 1977.

Leininger M: On open health care system model. *Nurs Outlook* 21:3:171-175, March 1973.

Lorig K: An overview of needs assessment tools for continuing education. *Nurs Educ* 2:2:12-16, March-April 1977.

Mayers M: *A Systematic Approach to the Nursing Care Plan.* 2nd ed, New York, Appleton-Century-Crofts, 1978.

McClure M: Entry into professional practice: The New York proposal. *J Nurs Adm* 6:5:12-17, June 1976.

Menke E: Theory development: A challenge for nursing. In Chaska N (ed): *The Nursing Profession: Views Through the Mist.* New York, McGraw-Hill Book Co, 1978, pp 216-221.

Mullane M: Roles and relationships: Nursing education. In Chaska N (ed): *The Nursing Profession: Views Through The Mist.* New York, McGraw-Hill Book Co, 1978, pp 37-42.

Nash G: Faculty evaluation. *Nurs Educ* 2:6:9-11, November-December 1977.

Ozimek D: *The Baccalaureate Graduate in Nursing, What Does Society Expect?* New York, National League for Nursing, 1974.

Redman B: Why develop a conceptual framework. *J Nurs Educ* 13:2-10, August 1974.

Ryan B: Nursing care plans: A systems approach to developing criteria for planning and evaluating. *J Nurs Adm* 3:3:50-73, May-June 1973.

Salk L, Kramer R: *How to Raise a Human Being.* New York, Random House, Inc. 1969.

Stevens, B: *The Nurse As Executive.* Wakefield, Mass, Contemporary Publishing Inc, 1975.

Styles M: In the name of integration. *Nurs Outlook* 24:12:738-744, December 1976.

Watson A, Mayers M: *Care Planning: Chronic Problem/Stat Solution.*Stockton, Calif, K/P Medical Systems, 1976.

Weiss C: Evaluation Research: Methods for Assessing Program Effectiveness. Englewood Cliffs, NJ, Prentice-Hall Inc, 1972.

Wong D: Providing experience in physical assessment for students in basic programs. *Am J Nurs* 75:6:974-975, June 1975.

Wyman J, Furnay K: Developing a criterion-referenced tool. *Nurs Outlook* 25:9:584-586, September 1977.

APPENDIX A
Assessment Guides:
Theories of Man

APPENDIX A
ASSESSMENT GUIDES: THEORIES OF MAN

Appendix A is a compilation of assessment guides. It is divided into six sections corresponding with the six systems of man: physiological, psychological, cognitive/intellectual, sensory/perceptive, interactive/affiliative, and mobile. Each section is preceded by an algorithm flow chart. The flow chart assumes that first- and second-level grand-tour questions have been asked and that a speculation has been made relative to which system or systems of man are probable problem areas. The flow chart uses Yes-No decision choices at several junctures, leading one either through a detailed assessment pathway (resulting in a nursing diagnosis) or through a pathway that bypasses detailed assessments, leading one to consider another system.

For the purposes of this text, assessment guides are not developed into finite detail. They are used to illustrate a process of using theories to develop assessment guides. Experts in any area of nursing can use a similar process to formulate algorithms allowing for in-depth assessment and specificity. Complete assessment questions, observations, and examinations have not been developed in this appendix for all the concepts, systems, and theories of man. Since the purpose of this text is to illustrate a process, the authors have used their own judgment to summarize theories, to interpret them, and to break them into theory elements, or criteria. This results in assessment guides which reflect the authors' arbitrary judgments.

Each algorithm is divided into one or more categories which have been derived from the major theories chosen to interpret a system of man. The assessment guides which appear after each algorithm chart state the major theory/s. The assessment guides appear as three-column charts. The first column shows theory elements labeled "Criteria". These are value-free terms. The second column, "Health Standards", converts the value-free term into a statement describing a desired level of performance with an assigned value. Column three depicts "Methods of Measurement: Questions, Observations and Inspections", designed to elicit data from which a judgment can be made relative to the Health Standard. The judgment is a nursing diagnosis. Chapter One details this decision process. Chapter Four explains how to use algorithms.

Physiological System Algorithm

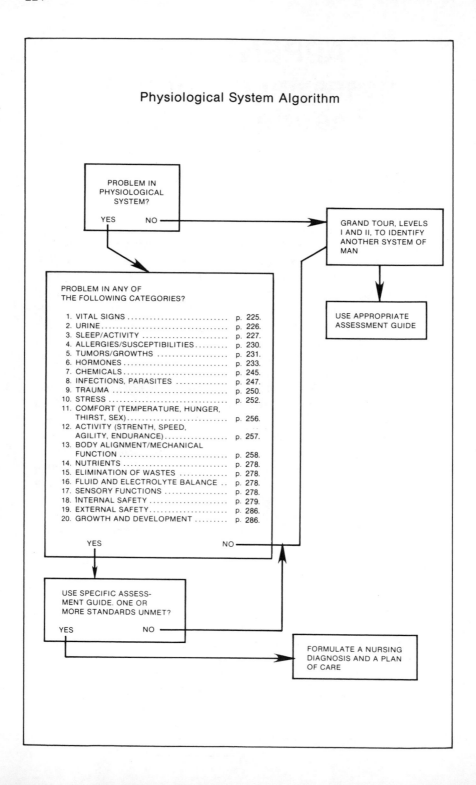

PROBLEM IN
PHYSIOLOGICAL
SYSTEM?

YES   NO

GRAND TOUR, LEVELS
I AND II, TO IDENTIFY
ANOTHER SYSTEM OF
MAN

PROBLEM IN ANY OF
THE FOLLOWING CATEGORIES?

1. VITAL SIGNS .... p. 225.
2. URINE.................................. p. 226.
3. SLEEP/ACTIVITY .... p. 227.
4. ALLERGIES/SUSCEPTIBILITIES......... p. 230.
5. TUMORS/GROWTHS .... p. 231.
6. HORMONES .... p. 233.
7. CHEMICALS............................ p. 245.
8. INFECTIONS, PARASITES .... p. 247.
9. TRAUMA .... p. 250.
10. STRESS .... p. 252.
11. COMFORT (TEMPERATURE, HUNGER,
    THIRST, SEX)........................... p. 256.
12. ACTIVITY (STRENTH, SPEED,
    AGILITY, ENDURANCE)................. p. 257.
13. BODY ALIGNMENT/MECHANICAL
    FUNCTION .... p. 258.
14. NUTRIENTS .... p. 278.
15. ELIMINATION OF WASTES .... p. 278.
16. FLUID AND ELECTROLYTE BALANCE .. p. 278.
17. SENSORY FUNCTIONS .... p. 278.
18. INTERNAL SAFETY .... p. 279.
19. EXTERNAL SAFETY..................... p. 286.
20. GROWTH AND DEVELOPMENT .... p. 286.

YES   NO

USE APPROPRIATE
ASSESSMENT GUIDE

USE SPECIFIC ASSESS-
MENT GUIDE. ONE OR
MORE STANDARDS UNMET?

YES   NO

FORMULATE A NURSING
DIAGNOSIS AND A PLAN
OF CARE

Physiological System

1. Vital Signs

CRITERIA	HEALTH STANDARDS	METHODS OF MEASUREMENT QUESTIONS, OBSERVATIONS, INSPECTIONS
Systems Theory: L. Bertalanffy[1] and Buckley[2] "...biologically life is not the maintenance of equilibrium but rather a dynamic dysequilibrium...to reach equilibrium (results in death)." Koestler, A. Man as a biological organism "contitutes a nicely integrated hierarchy of molecules, cells, organs, and organ systems."[3] Boulding — "Man as an open system maintains itself through import and export, building up and breaking down of its material components."[4]		
Physiological Parameters[5,6]	Capability of preventing injury or correcting damages.[5]	Take temperature at regular intervals at same level of activity each time. Use oral or rectal thermometer.
Temperature		
Oral	97-99.4° F or 36.1-37.4° C	
Rectal	98-100° F or 36.6-37.8° C	
Infant	No less than 96.9° F or 36.1° C	
Blood Pressure		Take blood pressure at regular intervals at same level of activity each time. Use stethoscope and sphygmomanometer.
Newborn (1-9 days)	56/40 mm. Hgb.	
Infant	78/40 mm. Hgb.	
Adolescent to middle adult	120/80 mm. Hgb.	
Older adult (60+)	140/90 mm. Hgb.	
Pulse, Apical	60-100 beats/minute	Count beats per minute at regular internals at same level of activity each time. Use stethoscope.

1. Vital Signs (cont.)

CRITERIA	HEALTH STANDARDS	METHODS OF MEASUREMENT QUESTIONS, OBSERVATIONS, INSPECTIONS
Skin color	Warm skin, no cyanosis	Inspect lips, nail beds and skin surfaces.
Respiratory rate and rhythm		Inspect chest, counting respirations per minute.
Newborn	30-80 breaths/minute	
Young child	20-40 breaths/minute	
Older child	15-25 breaths/minute	
Adult	16-22 breaths/minute	

Physiological System

2. Urine

CRITERIA	HEALTH STANDARDS	METHODS OF MEASUREMENT QUESTIONS, OBSERVATIONS, INSPECTIONS
Volume		Measure and record using a calibrated receptacle.
Newborn	30-60 ml./24 hours	
Infant		
3-10 days	100-300 ml./24 hours	
10 days-1 year	250-500 ml./24 hours	
Child		
1-5 years	500-700 ml./24 hours	
5-14 years	650-1400 ml./24 hours	
Adult, over 14 yr	600-1600 ml./24 hours	
Specific Gravity		Collect fresh specimens at specified intervals. Measure specific gravity with urinometer.

Newborn (1-2 days)	1.012	
Infant	1.002 - 1.006	
Adult	1.001 - 1.035	
pH	4.6 - 8.0	Dip litmus or nitrazine paper in fresh urine. Test area should be same color as normal range on chart.
Glucose	Negative	Dip glucose oxidase paper in fresh urine. Test area remains red.
Acetone	Negative	Use fresh urine, briefly dip reagent strip. Read in 15 seconds. Test area remains colorless.

Physiological System

3. Sleep and Activity

CRITERIA	HEALTH STANDARDS	METHOD OF MEASUREMENT QUESTIONS, OBSERVATIONS, INSPECTIONS
Sleep		Out of a twenty-four-hour period how many hours do you usually sleep.
Child	10-12 hours/24 hours	
Adult	6-9 hours/24 hours	at night?
Older Adult (60+)	Less than 6-8 hours/24 hours	during the day?
Activity		Observe in sleep and diaper change or ask mother or caretaker:
Infant 2 months	Moves often in sleep, wiggles when diaper changed.	Does child move during sleep and how much? Does he wiggle during diaper change?

3. Sleep and Activity *(cont.)*

CRITERIA	HEALTH STANDARDS	METHODS OF MEASUREMENT QUESTIONS, OBSERVATIONS, INSPECTIONS
6-9 months	Tries to stand and crawls.	Does child crawl? Does child attempt to crawl?
11-14 months	Walks alone, climbs, eats enthusiastically.	Does child walk without help? Does child try to climb? Does child like to eat?
Child		Describe child's eating habits.
2 year old	Explores, eats big lunch and bedtime snacks. Yells if feeling excitement or delight, cries if thwarted, runs to favorite people, resists strangers, resists going to bed.	How does child express excitement? What does child do if someone attempts to take toy away from him? What does child do when favorite family member enters the room?
5 year old	Always runs or walks fast; mastery of peddling performance; laughs a lot; smiles at everyone.	How easy is it for you to leave child with an unfamiliar person? Does your child go to bed easily? Does child hurry or take time to get places? Is child able to operate a tricycle? When child sees a cartoon on TV, what does he do? How friendly is he toward people?

3. Sleep and Activity (cont'd)

10-year-old	Participates in sports. Difficulty in sitting still.	Is child active in athletics? What sports does child prefer, if any?

Stage	Behavior	Questions
Early adolescent (Puberty 11-14)	Constantly interested in eating. Wants to stay up late at night. Boisterous, clumsy, aggressive behavior in boys. Play-acting, talkative, giggly behavior in girls.	How easy or hard is it for child to sit still long enough to accomplish homework, practice piano, attend a movie, etc.? Describe your eating habits. How late do you stay up at night? Describe typical behavior of child.
Late adolescent (15-19)	Participates in some physically active sport.	What, if any, sports are you active in?
Young Adult (20-30)	Enough energy to participate in leisure activities after completing necessary activities.	What leisure activities do you participate in? Do you have enough energy to do what you want to do? Do you have enough energy to do what you have to do?
Middle Adult (30-50)	Social activities decreasing; minimizing staying out late, particularly on work nights. Participation in fewer events than in early years. Patterns of work and leisure consistent with prior phase of life.	How much social activity do you participate in? How different is this from what you did ten to twelve years ago? How much time do you spend in leisure activities in relationship to work activities? Is "the above" the same as you did ten to fifteen years ago?

3. Sleep and Activity (cont.)

CRITERIA	HEALTH STANDARDS	METHODS OF MEASUREMENT QUESTIONS, OBSERVATIONS, INSPECTIONS
Middle Adult (50-70)	General decline in physical capacity and energy.	How busy is your life?
Old Adult (70+)	Participation in exercises beyond tasks of daily living.	Do you have the energy to do what you have to every day?
		Can you exceed minimal requirements? If yes, — daily?

Physiological System

4. Allergies and Susceptibilities

CRITERIA	HEALTH STANDARDS	METHODS OF MEASUREMENT QUESTIONS, OBSERVATIONS, INSPECTIONS
Immunological response	Ability to identify foreign materials causing physical discomfort.	What, if anything, are you allergic to: foods grasses molds dusts pollens animal danders serums

CRITERIA	HEALTH STANDARDS	METHODS OF MEASUREMENT QUESTIONS, OBSERVATIONS, INSPECTIONS
Resistance susceptibility cycle	Ability to plot energy cycles, plan activities according to cyclic rhythms.	vaccines drugs chemicals bee stings? Graph level of energy (low, medium, high) at hourly intervals for a twenty-four hour period. Graph energy cycle for longer period of time; week, month, season.

Physiological System

5. Tumors and Growths

CRITERIA	HEALTH STANDARDS	METHODS OF MEASUREMENT QUESTIONS, OBSERVATIONS, INSPECTIONS
Cell Division	No evidence of: Change in bowel or bladder habits. Sore that does not heal. Unusual bleeding or discharge. Thickening or lump in breast or elsewhere.	Have you had any: Change in bowel or bladder habits? Sore that does not heal? Unusual bleeding or discharge? Thickening or lump in breast or elsewhere?

5. Tumors and Growths *(cont.)*

CRITERIA	HEALTH STANDARDS	METHODS OF MEASUREMENT QUESTIONS, OBSERVATIONS, INSPECTIONS
	Indigestion or difficulty in swallowing.	Indigestion or difficulty in swallowing?
	Obvious change in wart or mole.	Obvious change in wart or mole?
	Nagging cough or hoarseness.	Nagging cough or hoarseness?
	No evidence of high risk: Family history of cancer.	Did anyone in your family have cancer or die of cancer?
	Personal past history of cancer.	Have you ever had any form of cancer?
	Employment in carcinogenic occupation.	Are you exposed to any of the following in daily life: radiation smokers dust or fibers in air (what kind)?
	Woman over age of 30-35. Man over age 40.	How old are you?

Physiological System

6. Hormones

CRITERIA	HEALTH STANDARDS	METHODS OF MEASUREMENT QUESTIONS, OBSERVATIONS, INSPECTIONS
Reciprocal Adaptation: Rogers, M.[8] and Dunn, H.[9] — Man is "perceived as... a set of interrelated parts which mutually react and maintain themselves by exchanging energy: Man transacts with other systems in his environment... the health status of an individual is seen by the interaction and integration of two ecological universes: The internal environment and the external environment in which he/she lives... and relates." "...a change in one part of a system will necessarily produce change in other parts of the system or systems."		
Chemical/hormonal agents[5]	Ability of the body's system to adapt to a particular environment.[5]	
	Normal regulatory receptors or awareness of malfunctions.	
	Ability to change the environment so as to adapt to physiological needs.[5]	
Internal agents	No evidence of thyroid imbalance.[11]	Do you to your knowledge have any problems with your thyroid being overactive (hyperthyroidism)?
	Answers consistent with accepted practice.	If yes, determine: Level of knowledge. Treatment regime.

6. Hormones (cont.)

CRITERIA	HEALTH STANDARDS	METHODS OF MEASUREMENT QUESTIONS, OBSERVATIONS, INSPECTIONS
		Rationale for treatment. Problems with managing regime.
	Ability to tolerate room temperatures.	If no, ask the questions below: Is it hard for you to tolerate heat and warm rooms?
		Have you noticed any change in your temperment — restlessness, irritability?
	Ease in swallowing.	Does your throat usually or ever feel full or swollen?
		Do you use iodized or noniodized salt?
		Have you ever lived in the Pacific Northwest or Great Lakes area?
		If so, for how long?
	Awareness of high risk.	If answer is yes to previous question, client is at high risk.
	Protrusion of eyeballs.	Inspect for exophthalmos.
	Thyroid not palpable or barely so without tenderness or nodules.[10]	Palpate thyroid.
		Do you to your knowledge have any problems with your thyroid being underactive (hypothyroidism)?

Answers consistent with accepted practice.	If yes, determine: Level of knowledge. Treatment regime. Rationale for treatment. Problems with managing regime. If no, ask the questions below:
Ability to tolerate cold.	Are you more sensitive to cold than you have been in the past?
Normal perspiration.	Do you perspire more or less than you used to?
Normally oily hair.	Would you say that your hair is basically dry or oily?
Ability to easily stay up past usual bedtime.	How early do you fall asleep in the evenings?
Normal bowel habits.	Do you have any trouble with constipation?
Normal weight for age and size.	Any weight gain?
	For women:
Normal menstrual period.	Have you had any menstrual disorder?
	For men:
Normal sexual pattern.	Have you experienced any change in your normal sex drive?

6. Hormones *(cont.)*

CRITERIA	HEALTH STANDARDS	METHODS OF MEASUREMENT QUESTIONS, OBSERVATIONS, INSPECTIONS
	No puffiness of hands, feet or eyes.	Is there puffiness of your hands, feet, or around your eyes?
	Normal hair condition.	Is you hair gradually thinning?
	Smooth, moist skin.	Inspect skin for roughness and hair for dryness.
	No evidence of insulin imblance.[11]	Do you to your knowledge have any symptoms of diabetes?
	Answers consistent with accepted practice.	If yes, determine: Level of knowledge. Treatment regimen. Rationale for treatment. Problem with managing regimen.
		If no, ask the questions below:
		Do you have a history of diabetes in your family?
		If a mother, have you every had a baby who weighed more than 9 lbs.?
	Awareness of high risk.	If answer to one or both of the two previous questions is yes, client is at high risk.
	Normal thirst.	Do you have any problems with feeling very thirsty,

voiding frequently in large amounts excessive appetite weight loss?

Normal urination.
Normal appetite.
Normal weight.

Do you ever have blurred vision?

Episodes of blurred vision.

Do you have any problems with skin infections or healing of infections?

Normal healing of lacerations or infections.

Measure height and weight.

Normal weight for height, sex and age.

Select random urine specimen and test for sugar and acetone with a uristick.

Negative uristick registers for sugar and acetone.

To your knowledge have you ever been told you have Addison's Disease, Cushing's Syndrome, or trouble with your adrenal glands?

No evidence of adrenal imbalance.[11]

If yes, determine:
Level of knowledge.
Treatment regimen.
Rationale for treatment.
Problems with managing regimen.

Answers consistent with accepted practice.

If no, ask the questions below:

Have you noticed:
Loss of strength.
Fatigue.
Loss of appetite.
Nausea/vomiting.
Abdominal pain.
Diarrhea.

Normal strength.
Minimal amounts of energy.
Normal appetite.
No nausea/vomiting.
No abdominal pain.
No diarrhea.

6. Hormones (cont.)

CRITERIA	HEALTH STANDARDS	METHODS OF MEASUREMENT QUESTIONS, OBSERVATIONS, INSPECTIONS
	No episodes of clustering of four symptoms; nervousness, headache, trembling, sweating.	Do you have episodes of nervousness, headaches, sweating, trembling?
	Normal muscular strength.	Have you noted any muscle wasting or weakness?
	Few, if any nose bleedings.	Do you have nosebleeds?
	Normal clotting when cut — normal bruises.	Do you bruise easily?
	Even temperament.	Do you feel irritable or have rapid mood changes?
	No swelling of ankles and legs.	Do you have a tendency for swelling of ankles and legs?
		Inspect for:
	No evidence of bronzing of skin in specified areas.	Bronze-like pigmentation of skin and mucous membranes.
	No evidence of hyperpigmentation of specified areas.	Hyperpigmentation of pressure points and elbows, knees and beltline.
	No evidence of buffalo hump, moon face, dispro-	Moon face. Accumulation of fat on face, back of neck

portion of fat on upper trunk.	and upper body. Purple striae on trunk and associated with obesity of trunk.
	To your knowledge have you ever been told you have a disease of the pituitary gland?
No evidence of pituitary imbalance.[11]	
Answers consistent with accepted practice.	If yes, determine: Level of knowledge. Treatment regime. Rationale for treatment. Problems with managing regime. If no, ask the questions below:
No evidence of visual disturbance.	Have you had any visual problems?
Freedom from severe headaches.	Have you had any severe headaches?
No observed changes in bones or joints.	Have you noticed any changes in your bones and joints — are they thicker, heavier, longer? Are your facial features about the same as they've always been or do they seem more coarse or heavy?
No alarming or radical change in glove and shoe size.	Have your glove and shoe sizes change?
No evidence of clustering of symptoms: Insatiable thirst.	Have you noticed an insatiable thirst, loss of appetite, weight loss and weakness?

6. Hormones *(cont.)*

CRITERIA	HEALTH STANDARDS	METHODS OF MEASUREMENT QUESTIONS, OBSERVATIONS, INSPECTIONS
	Anorexia. Weight loss. Weakness.	If adolescent, ask:
	Sexual development consistent with age and group referent.	Do you believe that you are as sexually developed as your peers?
	Development within normal ranges for height, weight and body configuation for age and sex.	If child, inspect for signs of dwarfism: shorter than average height for age; very small bone structure; immature body configuration for age.
	No evidence of:	If infant or young child, inspect for:
	Long wide bones.	Abnormally long and wide bones.
	Enlarged lower jaw.	Enlargement of lower jaw.
	Pronounced frontal sinuses.	Pronounced frontal sinuses.
	Wide large hands and feet.	Wide large hands and feet.
	Heavy lips and tongue.	Heavy lips and enlarged tongue.
	No evidence of genetic imbalance.[7]	To your knowledge have you ever been told you have sickle cell diseases or have your ever been told you have anemia?

Answers consistent with accepted practice.	If yes, determine: Level of knowledge. Treatment regime. Rationale for treatment. Problems with managing regime. If no, ask the questions below:
Absence of respiratory infections.	Do you have frequent respiratory infections including tonsillitis?
Absence of urinary tract infections.	Are you bothered by urinary tract infections?
Absence of infected sores.	Do you get infected sores on your legs?
No episodes of vomiting, diarrhea and polyuria.	Do you have episodes of vomiting, diarrhea and polyuria?
No bone and joint pain.	Do you have problems with bone and joint pain?
No jaundice.	Have you ever thought you had jaundice?
	Perform Sickledex text. Solution should remain clear after five minutes.
No evidence of enlarged lymph glands.	Palpate lymph glands at neck, axilla and groin.
No evidence of ocular lesions.	Examine eye grounds with otoscope. Look for ocular lesions such as retinal and vitreous hemorrhage, pigmented chorea, retinal lesions, tortuosity and dilatation of capillary bed, jaundice of eye sclera.

6. Hormones *(cont.)*

CRITERIA	HEALTH STANDARDS	METHODS OF MEASUREMENT QUESTIONS, OBSERVATIONS, INSPECTIONS
	Answers consistent with accepted practice.	To your knowledge have you ever been told you have hemophilia?
		If yes, determine:
		Level of knowledge. Treatment regime. Rationale for treatment. Problems with managing regime.
		If no, ask the questions below:
		Does anyone in your family have a history of hemophilia or bleeding?
		Do you have any history of renal, splenic or liver disease or some unusual bleeding problems?
		Do you for any reason frequently take aspirin or anticoagulants?
	Awareness of high risk.	If answer is yes to any of the 3 questions above, client is at high risk.
	Does not have frequent nosebleeds according to client's perception.	Do you have frequent nosebleeds?

Bleeding should stop within 3-8 minutes in adults.	If so, how long do they last? Have you had any recent bleeding that caused you alarm or would not stop?
Does not bruise easily according to perception of client.	Do you bruise easily?
Gums do not bleed.	Do your gums bleed when you brush your teeth?
No evidence of petechial ecchymosis in absence of severe blow to area.	Inspect body surfaces for petechial ecchymosis.
Liver edge should be firm, sharp, regular ridge with smooth surface. [10,12]	Palpate liver for structural characteristics.
	Has your child ever been diagnosed for cystic fibrosis?
	Has your baby (child) had any evidence of large, bulky, foul-smelling stools?
Answers consistent with accepted practice.	If yes, determine: Level of knowledge. Treatment regime. Rationale for treatment. Problems, if any, with managing regime. If no, ask the questions below:

6. Hormones *(cont.)*

CRITERIA	HEALTH STANDARDS	METHODS OF MEASUREMENT QUESTIONS, OBSERVATIONS, INSPECTIONS
	No evidence of coughing and sneezing.	Have you noticed a lot of coughing and sneezing (in child)?
	No evidence of salty residue on skin.	Have you noticed a salty taste on baby's skin when kissing baby?
	Weight within norms for age and sex.	Weigh.
	No evidence of protruberance of abdomen.	Inspect abdomen for protruberance.
	Normal muscular development of buttocks.	Inspect buttocks for wasted appearance.
	No evidence of wheezing, rales or dullness.	Auscultate chest for wheezing, rales or dullness.
	Stool should be normal bulk, color and odor without evidence of mucous.	Inspect stool, if available, for bulk, odor and mucous.
		Was your baby born in a hospital?
		Were you told by a doctor or nurse that your baby has PKU?
	Answers consistent with accepted practice.	If yes, determine: Level of knowledge.

Treatment regime.
Rationale for treatment.
Problems, if any, with managing regime.

If no, complete a Denver Development test.

Normal range for fine motor, gross motor and language.

Physiological System

7. Chemicals

CRITERIA	HEALTH STANDARDS	METHODS OF MEASUREMENT QUESTIONS, OBSERVATIONS, INSPECTIONS
External agents.	Answers represent no unusual hazard from poisons.	Where do you store your cleaning fluids and caustic material (poisons)?
		Does anyone in your family work with poisonous or highly caustic materials on their job?
	Answers represent no unusual hazard from drugs.	What drugs do you normally keep in your medicine chest?
	Awareness of high risk.	Are you allergic to any drug?
	Preventive measures used; e.g., Medic-Alert.	If answer is yes, client is at high risk.

7. Chemicals *(cont.)*

CRITERIA	HEALTH STANDARDS	METHODS OF MEASUREMENT QUESTIONS, OBSERVATIONS, INSPECTIONS
		Are there any other drugs which you use on social occasions such as: Alcohol Marijuana Cocaine LSD Coffee, tea, cocoa, cola drinks Cigarettes Glue Amphetamines Sedatives If answers yes to any of the drugs above, proceed to more specific questions such as those used by Alcoholics Anonymous, The Lung Association, a drug control center and those available in pharmacopeia.

Physiological System

8. Infections, Parasites

CRITERIA	HEALTH STANDARDS	METHODS OF MEASUREMENT QUESTIONS, OBSERVATIONS, INSPECTIONS
	Ability of the body's system to adapt to a particular microbiol invasion.	
	Ability to manipulate the environment to reduce the potential for microbiol parasitic invasion.	
	Absence of discharge and sores in the genital area.	Do you or any members of your family have any problems with discharges or sores in the genital area; urinary tract infections (venereal disease)?
		Have you or anyone in your family in the last year or two had problems of this nature?
		If no, go no further.
		If yes, ask client to describe and be specific.
	Answers consistent with accepted practice.	What do you know about the current prevalence of venereal diseases; how they are transmitted; what problems they cause?

8. Infections, Parasites *(cont.)*

CRITERIA	HEALTH STANDARDS	METHODS OF MEASUREMENT QUESTIONS, OBSERVATIONS, INSPECTIONS
	Documented evidence of immunization according to State standards.	When were you and/or members of your family last immunized for: Measles Mumps Poliomyelitis Diphtheria Whooping Cough Tetanus Smallpox?
		Have you ever been told that you have liver disease or trouble with your spleen (or spleen removed)?
	Documented evidence of immunization to: Pneumocci Flu Other microbes	If yes, ask client to describe and be specific. Have you or anyone in your family, or close friend ever been told they have tuberculosis?
	Answers consistent with accepted practice.	If yes, determine: Level of knowledge. Treatment regime. Rationale for treatment. Problems, if any, with managing regime.

In presence of high-risk factors, x-ray or skin test done within last year.	How recently have you or other members of your family had either a chest x-ray or skin test for tuberculosis? In high risk infants (low socioeconomic, under age six months) inspect for Shigellosis.
Normal elasticity of skin.	Check skin turgor.
No evidence of wasting of subcutaneous tissue.	
Formed or semi-formed stool — no evidence of watery mucous.	Collect stool specimen.
Temperature below 99.8°R.	Measure temperature.
Normal activity for age.	Observe activity level.
No evidence of numerous fleas.	Observe sanitation of environment.
Evidence of handwashing facilities and refrigeration.	

Physiological System

9. Trauma

CRITERIA	HEALTH STANDARDS	METHODS OF MEASUREMENT QUESTIONS, OBSERVATIONS, INSPECTIONS
Traumatic agents	Ability to manipulate the environment to reduce the potential for traumatic injury. Ability to repair damages received by trauma.	
Human	No evidence of abuse in prior or present generation.	Can you recall hearing of any physical abuses in your family: Child abuse, physical or psychological? Husband abuse? Wife abuse? Sexual abuse? Observe for nonverbal expressions of fear when question asked. Inspect for obvious physical trauma such as bruises, swollen limbs and lacerations.
	Answers should be consistent with current recommendations for safety:	Do you feel you are physically at risk with other people?

	Locking devices, concealing purses.	Robbery?
	Rape prevention.	Rape?
	Defensive driving, walking, biking and boating.	Motoring? Sports?
	Avoiding high crime area.	Vandalism?
		If so, what mechanisms can you use to avoid harm?
	Awareness of the client when he is at risk for self-harm:	What mechanisms can you use to avoid self-injury?
	Psychologically stressed	
	Fatigued	
	Chronically ill	
	History of accident proneness	
Non-human	Absence of harmful elements.	Observe for:
	Litter	Litter and clutter
	Furniture	Unsafe furniture
	Unsafe floors	Unsafe floors — slippery, uneven
	Lighting	Inadequate lighting
	Electrical devices	Unsafe electrical practices
	Thermal dangers	Thermal dangers
		Hot water
		Fire hazards

Physiological System

10. Stress

CRITERIA	HEALTH STANDARDS	METHODS OF MEASUREMENT QUESTIONS, OBSERVATIONS, INSPECTIONS
Stress Theory: Selye — "Man responds to stress of any kind with a unified defense mechanism characterized by specific structural and chemical changes. This reaction can raise the body's resistance to stressful agents and can also be used to protect against disease. But when the reaction is faulty or overly prolonged, it can also produce disease or even death."[13]		
Selye's theory is referred to as the General Adaptation Syndrom (GAS) which includes alarm reaction, stage of resistance and state of exhaustion.[14]		
Physiological responses[15,12]	Ability of the body to mobilize temporary defense forces.	Inspect laboratory values:
Alarm Reaction		
Sodium chloride level of the blood.	Decreased sodium chloride level in extra-cellular fluid, chloride approximately 96 mEq/L; sodium 135 mEq/L sodium.	Serum chloride and sodium.
Blood potassium.	Increased blood potassium approximately or above 5 mEq/L.	Serum potassium.

Blood glucose.	Decreased blood glucose followed by increased blood glucose level (Folin); decreased 80 mg/100 ml. followed by increased 120 mg/100 ml.	Fasting blood glucose.
	Evidence of:	Inspect or observe:
	Pale skin	Skin
	Cool moist skin	
	Dilated pupils	Pupils
	Tense muscles	Muscles
	Keen mental alertness	Mentation
	Full, rapid pulse	Pulse
	Elevated systolic blood pressure.	Blood pressure
	Deep respiration	Respirations
Stage of Resistance	Ability of the organism to maintain adaptation to a stressor.	Inspect laboratory values for:
ACTH secretions	Increased ACTH secretions measured by 17 ketosteroids: 4-18 mg/24 hours urine; 125 mcg/100 ml. in blood plasma.	Urine — 17 ketosteroids.
	Blood values return to normal.	

10. Stress (cont.)

CRITERIA	HEALTH STANDARDS	METHODS OF MEASUREMENT QUESTIONS, OBSERVATIONS, INSPECTIONS
	Serum chloride — 96-106 mEq/liter.	Serum chloride and sodium.
	Serum sodium — 136-145 mEq/liter.	
	Serum potassium — 3.5-5.0 mEq/liter.	Serum potassium.
	Blood glucose — fasting 80-120 mg/100 ml.	Blood glucose.
Psychological response[16]	Evidence of: Distractable behavior. Frustration Masking of motives Masking of anxiety Distorting: Perception Memory Action Motivation Thought	Observe adaptive mechanisms.

Stage of Exhaustion[17]		Inspect:
	Ability to remove or diminish the stressor before exhaustion occurs.	
	No evidence of:	
	Cyanosis or ashen color. Cold perspiration.	Skin
	Dilated pupils.	Pupils
	Lethargy or flaccid muscles.	Muscles
	Weak, thready, rapid, irregular pulse.	Apical pulse
	Drowsiness, slowed re-action time, intermittent consciousness, un-consciousness.	
	Decreased systolic or diastolic blood pressure.	Blood pressure
	Shallow, rapid respirations.	
	Urinary output of less than 15 cc/hour.	Urinary output

Physiological System

11. Comfort (Hunger, Thirst, Temperature, Sex)

Growth and Development: Maslow, A. Maslow's hierarchy identifies five levels of human needs. The first two needs, physiological and safety, relate to Man as a physiological system. Physiological needs include hunger, thirst, shelter, sex, and other needs. Safety includes security and protection from physical...harm."[18]

CRITERIA	HEALTH STANDARDS	METHODS OF MEASUREMENT QUESTIONS, OBSERVATIONS, INSPECTIONS
Physiological Needs	Perceived satisfaction of basic physiological needs.	
Comfort	Hunger	Are you able to get food when you feel hungry?
		What kinds of foods satisfy your hunger?
	Thirst	Are you able to get something to drink when you feel thirsty?
		What kinds of liquids satisfy your thirst?
	Sex	Are you able to satisfactorily relieve physical sexual tension?
	Warmth	Does your home or work environment satisfactorily protect you from the outside elements:
		Heat?
		Cold?
		Snow, rain?
		Sun?
		Wind?
		Do your clothes and blankets keep you comfortable?

Physiological System

12. Activity (Strength, Speed, Agility, Endurance)

CRITERIA	HEALTH STANDARDS	METHODS OF MEASUREMENT QUESTIONS, OBSERVATIONS, INSPECTIONS
Activity	Ability to meet necessary activities of daily living.	What are those activities (sports, exercises, work, social) that you engage in?
Strength Speed Agility Endurance		Do you find that you have enough physical strength for these activities?
		Are your endurance levels adequate to meet the demands of these activities?
Cardiac tolerance	State of activity which does not exceed cardiac tolerance levels. In absence of known cardiac problems: Under age 30, pulse rate should not exceed 151 ten seconds after performing calisthenics.[19] Over age 30, pulse rate should not exceed 131 ten seconds after performing calisthenics.	Inspect for cardiac tolerance by having person do a selected type of calisthenics, then checking pulse ten seconds afterwards.

Physiological System

13. Body Alignment/Mechanical Function

CRITERIA	HEALTH STANDARDS	METHODS OF MEASUREMENT QUESTIONS, OBSERVATIONS, INSPECTIONS
Body alignment and mechanical function.	Structural, muscular and mechanical correlation that allows for necessary mobility.[19]	
Structure	When standing:	Inspect and observe:
	Head, upper torso and lower torso should be in line with one another.	Front and back views of undressed body.
	Shoulders and iliac crest should be parallel in height.	Front and back views of undressed body.
	Spine should not be curved laterally.	Back view of undressed body.
	There should be no exaggerated flattening of curvature of lumbar spine.	Side view of undressed body.
	There should not be exaggerated rounding of thoracic spine.	Side view of undressed body.

Musculature[20]	When lying: Body relationships should be the same as when standing. Presence of muscle, bulk: Body contour should be consistent with normal figure of like sex and age. Size, contour and strength should be symmetrical on each side of body. Difference of 1 cm. not significant.	Supine, side-lying and prone body positions. Inspect and compare client's body against a body contour image. Position body in supine position — observe for symmetry. Inspect muscle contours during contraction and rest. If asymmetry suspected, measure circumferences bilaterally at maximum girth.
Muscle tone	Evidence of mild, even muscle resistance "when relaxed limb is passively moved through range of motion."[20] "Normal limbs swing freely in a regular pendulum-like motion, decreasing in a steady, even manner."[20]	Move each limb through flexion, extension and rotation, both rapidly and slowly. Flip client's arms out from hips and allow them to drop. While client is sitting, raise his legs and allow them to drop.
Muscle strength[20]	Smooth, steady counter-pressure as joint is moved.	Perform muscle strength test:

13. Body Alignment/Mechanical Function (cont.)

CRITERIA	HEALTH STANDARDS	METHODS OF MEASUREMENT QUESTIONS, OBSERVATIONS, INSPECTIONS
		Neck:
		Flexion and extension.
		Ask client to put chin on chest and then move head backwards as far as possible. During his movement, examiner puts finger-tips against forehead and palm of hand against occiput.
		Fingers:
		Flexion
		Ask client to squeeze examiner's fingers hard and to make a fist. Examiner resists by gripping, attempting to withdraw and straighten his fingers.
		Extension
		Have client hold fingers out straight. Examiner attempts finger flexion.
		Adduction
		Client holds paper between adjacent fingers. Examiner pulls paper.
		Abduction
		Client holds fingers straight out and spread apart. Examiner attempts to squeeze adjacent fingers together.

Wrist:

Flexion

Client flexes wrist and examiner tries
to extend wrist.

Extension

Client pronates forearm and cocks up
wrist. Examiner presses dorsum of hand
to push wrist down.

Elbow:

Flexion (Biceps)

Client flexes elbow 90° and attempts to
bend more. Examiner prevents flexion.

Supination and Pronation

(Palm up) Client rotates wrist in one
direction then the other. Examiner resists
efforts to rotate.

Extension (Triceps)

Client flexes elbow to varying degrees and
attempts to straighten. Examiner prevents
straightening.

Shoulder:

Abduction (Deltoid)

Client holds upper arm out horizontally.
Examiner attempts to depress elbow.

13. Body Alignment/Mechanical Function (cont.)

CRITERIA	HEALTH STANDARDS	METHODS OF MEASUREMENT QUESTIONS, OBSERVATIONS, INSPECTIONS
		Adduction
		Client holds upper arm close to chest. Examiner attempts to raise elbow horizontally.
		Ankle:
		Dorsi-flexion
		Client walks on heels and pulls foot and toes upward. Examiner pushes downward on foot.
		Plantar-flexion
		Client walks on toes and pushes down as examiner pushes up against bottom of foot.
		Knee:
		Flexion (Hamstring)
		Client sits bending knee at 90° angle, tries to flex further. Examiner resists further flexion.
		Extension (Quadriceps)
		Client squats and arises while examiner pushes down to prevent knee flexion.

Hip:

Flexion

Client sits raising knee upward while examiner pushes downward directly above knee.

Extension

Client ascends a step, rising from squatting position.

Abduction

Client holds knees tightly together. Examiner tries to separate knees.

Trunk:

Abdomen

Client rises from lying to sitting position.

Back

Client lies on side or in prone position and elevates leg or head.

Inspect main joints.

90°

FLEXION

150°

180°

0°

NEUTRAL
10°

HYPEREXTENSION

From Joint Motor Manual, Courtesy of American Academy of Orthopedic Surgeons.

Mechanical joint motion and function

Joints should move in directions and to the degree as that typical of person of same age and sex.[10]

13. Body Alignment/Mechanical Function (cont.)

CRITERIA	HEALTH STANDARDS	METHODS OF MEASUREMENT QUESTIONS, OBSERVATIONS, INSPECTIONS
		Test for joint mobility:
		Wrist:
	Normal range — radial deviation 20° to ulnar deviation 55°	Abduction and Adduction
		Place hand in flat horizontal (0 degree) position. Have client move hand from wrist as far to right and to the left as possible.
	Normal range — extension to 70° from 0 flexion to 90° from 0.	Extension and Flexion
		Client holds hand horizontally, freely in air. Ask client to extend from wrist as far as possible and to flex from wrist as far as possible.
		Elbow:
	Normal range — supination 90° from 0, pronation 90° from 0.	Supination and Pronation
		Have client close fist and place arm on table directly in front. Ask client to rotate from elbow as far as possible to the left and to the right.
	Normal range — flexion 160° from 0, extension 0.	Flexion and Extension

Client to stand with arms straight at sides, palms facing forward. Ask client to raise hand from elbow as far as possible, keeping wrist straight.

Shoulder:

Abduction and Adduction

Ask client to stand facing examiner. From shoulder, hold arm straight out from body, wrist straight, palms downward. Ask client to move arm as high as possible in passing in front of body.

Normal range — abduction 180° from 0, adduction 50°

Internal and external rotation

Ask client to stand with lateral view to examiner, hold upper arm straight out from body, elbow flexed to 90° at same level, palm downward.

Normal range internal 90° from 0; external 90° from 0.

Internal

Ask client to move arm from shoulder in a downward arc, as far as possible.

External

From 0 position, ask client to move arm from shoulder in an upward arc, as far as possible.

266

13. Body Alignment/Mechanical Function (cont.)

CRITERIA	HEALTH STANDARDS	METHODS OF MEASUREMENT QUESTIONS, OBSERVATIONS, INSPECTIONS
	Normal range extension 50° from 0; flexion 180° from 0.	Extension and flexion Ask client to stand with lateral view to examiner. Ask him to hold arm straight out in front of body, elbow straight, wrist straight, palms down. Ask client to move arm in an arc as far as possible (extension) and to move arm upward from shoulder as high as possible (flexion).
		Ankles and Feet:
	Normal range 20° from 0; Plantar flexion 45° from 0.	Dorisflexion and plantar flexion With client in supine position, place ankle in 0 position (90° flexion). From this position, ask client to flex ankle as far as possible toward body (dorsi-flexion) and to straighten ankle away from body as far as possible (plantar flexion).
	Normal range — inversion 50° from 0; eversion 20° from 0.	Inversion and eversion Have client stand barefoot, facing examiner. Ask client to lift inside of foot as far as possible, leaving outside

of foot on floor (inversion). Then ask client to elevate outside of foot as far as possible keeping inside of foot on floor (eversion).

Knees:

Extension and flexion

Have client in supine position with body supported to mid thigh. Ask client to raise leg from knee as far as possible (hyperextension). Ask client to lower leg in an arc downward and as far back as possible (flexion).

Hypertension to 15° from 0; flexion 130° from 0.

Hips:

Hyperextension and flexion

Have client lie in supine position with body supported to mid hip line, legs straight, ankle flexed to 90°. Ask client to move leg downward from hip as far as possible (hyperextension). Then ask him to raise his leg from the hip as far as possible keeping knee straight and ankle flexed.

With knee straight, hyperextension 15° from 0; flexion 90° from 0.

13. Body Alignment/Mechanical Function *(cont.)*

CRITERIA	HEALTH STANDARDS	METHODS OF MEASUREMENT QUESTIONS, OBSERVATIONS, INSPECTIONS
	With knee flexed, Extension 0° and flexion 120° from 0.	Extension and flexion Have client lie in supine position. Ask client to rest knee flat on surface (extension). Ask client to bring knees as close to abdomen as possible keeping knee flexed (flexion).
	Abduction — 45° from 0. Adduction — 30° from 0.	Abduction and adduction Have client stand facing examiner, feet slightly apart. Ask client to move leg outward keeping knee straight (abduction). Then ask him to move leg across front of opposite leg as far as possible, keeping knee straight (adduction).
	Internal — 40° from 0. External — 45° from 0.	Internal and external rotation Ask client to stand facing examiner. Ask him to bring knee to 90° angle from body with lower leg hanging freely downward in front. Ask client to rotate leg from hip outward as far as possible (internal rotation). Then from same 0 position, rotate leg inward past front of other leg as far as possible (external rotation).

Cervical spine:

Extension and flexion

Have client assume a position in lateral views to examiner with neck in 0 position (in straight alignment with shoulders). From that position ask client to move head backwards as far as possible, bending at neck (extension). From 0 position, ask client to move head forward or downward as far as possible, bending at neck (flexion).

Extension — 55° from 0.
Flexion — 45° from 0.

Lateral bending

Have client face examiner, holding head and neck in 0 position (straight alignment with rest of body). Ask client to move head, bending at neck to the right and to the left as far as possible.

Right 40° from 0.
Left 40° from 0.

Rotation

Have client lie in supine position, shoulders flat on examining surface, with head and neck in straight alignment with rest of body (0 position). From this position, ask client to turn his head as far as possible to the right and to the left.

Right 70° from 0.
Left 70° from 0.

13. Body Alignment/Mechanical Function (cont.)

CRITERIA	HEALTH STANDARDS	METHODS OF MEASUREMENT QUESTIONS, OBSERVATIONS, INSPECTIONS
		Lumbo-sacral spine:
	Extension 30° from 0. Flexion 75° to 90° from 0.	Extension and flexion
		Have client assume a standing lateral position to examiner. Ask client to bend from hips backward as far as possible (extension). Then to bend forward from hips as far as possible, keeping knees straight (flexion).
		Lateral bending
	Right 35° from 0. Left 35° from 0.	Have client stand with back to examiner in 0 position. Ask him to bend, keeping hips flexed as far to the right and as far to the left as possible.
		Rotation
	Right 30° from 0. Left 30° from 0.	Have client assume supine position with hips stabilized. Ask him to rotate right side of upper torso downward as far as possible and repeat on the left side.
Reflexes[20]	Presence of reflexes	Test for reflexes
	Extension of arm	Triceps

	Place client in sitting position, examiner supporting arm at wrist. Strike tendon with reflex hammer directly above elbow.
	Brachio-radialis
Flexion of forearms and fingers.	Have client assume recumbent position. Place hands on abdomen. Strike client's forearm with reflex hammer midway between shoulder and elbow.
	Quadriceps (knee jerk)
Quadriceps contraction and knee extension.	Have client assume sitting position with legs dangling knees apart. Strike tendon just below patella.
	Achilles (ankle jerk)
Plantar flexion	Have client sit or lie in supine position. Place gentle pressure on ball of foot. Strike across tendon with reflex hammer.
	Jaw
Closure of jaw.	Have client relax jaw, partially opened. Examiner presses downward with one finger on the chin. Tap finger with reflex hammer.
	Babinsky
Plantar flexion of toes.	Have client assume relaxed recumbent position with legs extended. Examiner then

13. Body Alignment/Mechanical Function *(cont.)*

CRITERIA	HEALTH STANDARDS	METHODS OF MEASUREMENT QUESTIONS, OBSERVATIONS, INSPECTIONS
		applies a firm stroke with a key or orange stick against sole of foot. The stroke begins at the lateral aspect of the heel, is moved slowly upward toward little toe and across ball of foot toward large toe.
Coordination	Presence of coordination[20]	Test for coordination
	Smooth movements and maintenance of body posture.	Finger to nose Have client sit with arms extended forward, touching nose with a forefinger, returning arm to extended position. Do both with eyes open and with eyes closed.
	Ability to touch four fingers on first try with smooth movements.	Four-finger approximation Have client extend arms out at sides, bringing them foward until four fingers meet at the midline. Do this first with eyes open and then with eyes closed.
	Maintenance of balance without shifting feet.	Romberg's sign Ask client to walk, first naturally, then in tandem fashion, placing the heel directly in front of the toe. Do this with eyes open and closed.

Chest topography[10,20,22]	Structure of chest and heart adequate for respiratory and circulatory function.	Inspect chest by observing, palpating, percussing and auscultating.
		Posterior Chest:
		From midline position behind the client (undressed to waist), examiner looks for the following:
	Chest should be symmetrical.	Deformities of thorax.
	Ribs should slope downward from midline.	Slope of ribs.
	Absence of retraction during inspiration. Absence of bulging during expiration.	Retraction of interspaces during inspiration. Ask client to breathe in and out several times, observing interspaces.
	Presence of normal respiratory excursion (free, even, symmetrical chest movement).	Respiratory rate and rhythm by examiner placing thumbs at about the level of and parallel to the 10th ribs, grasping the lateral rib cage. Ask client to inhale deeply.
	Fremitus (vibrations) should be present over each palpated area.	Examiner uses ball of hand over five bilateral areas of the posterior chest, asking the client to repeat the words "99" or "111".
	Resonance present at every point.	Using percussion techniques, percuss symmetrical areas at about 5 cm. areas down chest wall bilaterally.

13. Body Alignment/Mechanical Function (cont.)

CRITERIA	HEALTH STANDARDS	METHODS OF MEASUREMENT QUESTIONS, OBSERVATIONS, INSPECTIONS
	Breath sounds present at each auscultation point.	Using stethoscope, listen to client's lungs as he breathes through his mouth more deeply than normal. Listen to at least one full breath, moving downward on chest at 5 cm. intervals on chest wall bilaterally.
		Anterior chest:
		Repeat inspection for posterior chest, inspection, palpation, percussion and auscultation.
Heart function	Mechanical function of heart is within normal limits.	Inspect heart by observing, palpating, percussing and auscultating.
		With ball of hand, palpate the following areas:
	Aortic absence of pulsation, thrill or vibration.	Aortic — second interspace to right of sternum.
	Pulmonary absence of pulsation, thrill or vibration.	Pulmonary — second left interspace followed by third left interspace.
	Ventricular absence of diffuse lift or heave or thrills.	Right ventricular — lower half of sternum.
	Apical — presence of	Apical — or left ventricular — 5th

	intercostal or medial, to midclavicular line.	light tap at apical beat and absence of thrills or extra impulses.
	Epigastric — lower end of sternum, sliding fingers up under ribcage.	Epigastric — should feel aortic pulsation against palmar surface of finger and right ventricle beating downward against fingertips.
	Examiner, using percussion technique, moves at 1 cm. intervals laterally to medially in 3rd, 4th and 5th interspaces, listens for dullness indicating edge of heart.	Heart should be 4, 7, and 10 cm. in each of three interspaces respectively measuring distance from midsternal line.
	Check rate and rhythm using auscultation techniques, count rate per minutes: Aortic area Pulmonic area Ecke's point Tricuspid area Mitral area	At each point, regular beat and absence of intensity or splitting of first heart sounds. No extra sounds in systole or diastole. No systolic or diastolic murmur.
Vascular function	Inspect for vascular perfusion and structure through observing and palpating.	Presence of normal peripheral vascular perfusion. Evidence of normal vascular structure.

13. Body Alignment/Mechanical Function (cont.)

CRITERIA	HEALTH STANDARDS	METHODS OF MEASUREMENT QUESTIONS, OBSERVATIONS, INSPECTIONS
		Upper extremity:
	Veins of hand and forearm appear dilated when hand below heart and collapse within a few seconds when extremity is raised.	Client holds hand below level of heart, then raises arm to a 30° angle.
	Arterial pulses should be strong, equal in quality at time of arrival at examiner's fingertips.	Take radial arterial pulses bilaterally and simultaneously.
		Lower extremity:
	No evidence of obviously dilated or tortuous veins.	Inspect for varicose veins or edema.
	No evidence of edema.	
	Arterial pulses should be strong, equal in quality and time of arrival at examiner's fingertips.	Palpate femoral, dorsalis pedis and posterior tibial arteris bilaterally, simultaneously.
		Capillary perfusion:
	Absence of dusky, bluish coloration.	Inspect for general facial color especially about lips.

Absence of drawn, anxious expression.	Observe facial expression.
Able to talk continuously without gasping.	Count number of words client can say before gasping for breath.
Absence of vertical ridging of fingernails.	Inspect fingers and fingernails.
Absence of dusky, bluish coloration, immediate blotching and immediate return to normal color.	Pinch nail beds and observe for return of normal color.

Physiological System
14. Nutrients
15. Elimination of Wastes
16. Fluid and Electrolyte Balance
17. Sensory Functions

CRITERIA	HEALTH STANDARDS	METHOD OF MEASUREMENT QUESTIONS, OBSERVATIONS, INSPECTIONS
14. Nutrients		In a complete assessment guide, for each of the criteria elements listed in the left-hand column, similar details for the remaining columns would be included. For the purposes of this book these criteria elements have not been developed in detail.
15. Elimination of Wastes		
16. Fluid and electrolyte balance		
17. Sensory Functions		

Physiological System
18. Internal Safety

CRITERIA	HEALTH STANDARDS	METHODS OF MEASUREMENT QUESTIONS, OBSERVATIONS, INSPECTIONS
Safety needs	Perceived sense of security and freedom from threat.	
Physiological integrity		General status

Feelings of strength and vigor.	Are you feeling any concern about the following:
	Weakness
Enough energy to do what client desires.	Fatigue
Normal temperature.	Fever
	Chills
Warm moist skin.	Profuse perspiration
Absence of night sweats.	Night sweats
Normal weight for age and sex.	Weight changes
	Take temperature and weigh.
No evidence of irregular skin conditions:	Skin
	Do any of the following symptoms remind you of any concerns or fears you might have?
Itching	Itching
Color changes	Color changes
Texture changes	Texture changes
Temperature changes	Temperature changes
Excessive moisture or dryness	Excessive moisture or dryness
Bruises	Bruises
Petechiae	Petechiae

18. Internal Safety *(cont.)*

CRITERIA	HEALTH STANDARDS	METHODS OF MEASUREMENT QUESTIONS, OBSERVATIONS, INSPECTIONS
	Changes in birthmarks or moles.	Changes in birthmarks or moles.
	Changes in bodily hair.	Changes in bodily hair.
	Changes in fingernails (brittleness, ridging or pitting).	Changes in fingernails (brittleness, ridging or pitting).
	Rashes Hives Infections Delayed healing of a wound.	Rashes Hives Infections Delayed healing of a wound.
		Inspect integumentary surfaces
	Skin tests, injections, vaccinations, immunizations or desensitizations for pre-ventative reasons only?	Have you had any of the following? If so, why? Skin tests Injections Vaccinations Immunizations Desensitizations
		Head and face
	No evidence of the following:	Do any of the following symptoms remind you of fears or concerns that you have now or have had in the past?

Headaches
Facial pain
Dizziness
Fainting
Seizures
Trauma

Eyes

Are you having any of the following eye symptoms:

Pain
Sensitivity to light
Itching
Burning
Blindness
Double vision
Excessive tearing
Difficulty in seeing
Wearing of glasses
Date of last eye test
Infection
Glaucoma
Cataract
Foreign body
Operation

Perform visual acuity test using Snellen chart.

Perform funduscopic examination with ophthalmoscope.

Headaches
Facial pain
Dizziness
Fainting
Seizures
Trauma

Absence or nonpathological explanation for presence of:

Pain
Sensitivity to light
Itching
Burning
Blindness
Double vision
Excessive tearing
Difficulty in seeing
Wearing of glasses
Date of last eye test
Infection
Glaucoma
Cataract
Foreign body
Operation

At least 20/40 vision[12]

Eye disc should be round or vertically oval, paler or

18. Internal Safety (cont.)

CRITERIA	HEALTH STANDARDS	METHODS OF MEASUREMENT QUESTIONS, OBSERVATIONS, INSPECTIONS
	pinker than surrounding retinal tissue, located slightly to nasal side of center of retina. Disc is flat or slightly depressed, sharply defined edges. Arteries and veins should be spread out from disc in softly curving lines without evidence of hemorrhages.[12]	
		Ears
		Do any of the following cause you concerns?
	Absence of or nonpathological explanation for: Earache Itching Drainage Ringing of ears Difficulty in hearing Infections Foreign body Operation/s	Earache Itching Drainage Ringing of ears Difficulty in hearing Infections Foreign body Operation/s
	Eardrum should be shiny and pearly gray in color with no purulent discharge.	Inspect ear with otoscope.

Perform Rinne's test and Weber test with tuning fork.[12]

Nose and sinuses

Do you have or have you had any difficulties with the following:

Sinus pain?
Nose bleeds?
Nasal obstruction?
Nasal discharge?
Post-nasal drip?
Sneezing?
Change in sense of smell?
Frequent colds?
Allegic rhinitis
Foreign body
Operation/s

Inspect nose for:

Color of nasal mucosa

Septal deviation

Polyps

Mouth, Pharynx, Larynx

Eardrum should be slightly concave.

Sound should be heard equally in both ears.

Absence of or nonpathological explanation for:

Sinus pain
Nose bleeds
Nasal obstruction
Nasal discharge
Post-nasal drip
Sneezing
Change in sense of smell
Frequent colds
Allergic rhinitis
Foreign body
Operation/s

Nasal mucosa should be pink, not red, edematous, pale or boggy.

Absence of septal deviation with no more than slight decline.

No evidence of polyps.

18. Internal Safety (cont.)

CRITERIA	HEALTH STANDARDS	METHODS OF MEASUREMENT QUESTIONS, OBSERVATIONS, INSPECTIONS
	Absence of or nonpatholog-ical explanation for:	Do you have any concerns about any of the following:
	Sore tongue	Sore tongue?
	Tender gums	Tender gums?
	Toothache	Toothache?
	Mucosal erosions	Mucosal erosions?
	Bleeding gums	Bleeding gums?
	Tooth abscess	Tooth abscess?
	Tooth extractions	Tooth extractions?
	Dentures	Dentures?
	Too much or too little salivation	Too much or too little salivation?
	Changes in ability to taste	Changes in ability to taste?
	Sore throat	Sore throat?
	Difficulty in swallowing	Difficulty in swallowing?
	Hoarseness	Hoarseness?
	Infection	Infection?
	Operation	Operation?
		Inspect oral cavity for:
	Absence of or repaired caries.	Caries
	Pink firm gums.	Peridontal disease

Buccal mucosa/color

Tongue

Inspect for:

Size

Color

Surface characteristics

Movement

No evidence of red
swellings or gums
receding from teeth.

Buccal mucosa should
be smooth and pink. No
evidence of pallor,
yellow discoloration,
dusky blue cast,
melanotic spots.

Size normal for age.

Pink, no evidence
marked reddening or
thick white coating.

No evidence of deep
longitudinal fissures.

No evidence of sores or
tumors.

No evidence of tremor
or lateral deviation.

Other physiological parameters would be similarly developed for assessment of:

Neck   Gastrointestinal System
Endocrine System   Urinary System
Breasts   Reproductive System
Respiratory System   Skeletal System
Blood   Nervous System

Physiological System
19. External Safety

CRITERIA	HEALTH STANDARDS	METHODS OF MEASUREMENT QUESTIONS, OBSERVATIONS, INSPECTIONS
Safety Needs Environmental Chemical Microbial/Parasitic Traumatic (Mechanical)	See standards and data collection methods under Theory of Reciprocal Adaptation, Physiological Algorithms 7, 8 and 9.	

Physiological System
20. Growth and Development

Tanner, J. and Taylor, G. — Growth is "the series of orderly and irreversible stages that every organism goes through from the beginning of its life to the end."[23]

CRITERIA	HEALTH STANDARDS	METHODS OF MEASUREMENT QUESTIONS, OBSERVATIONS, INSPECTIONS
Growth and development norms for: Weight Height Activity Developmental tasks	In a complete assessment guide, for each of the criteria elements listed in the left-hand column, details for the remaining columns would be included. For the purposes of this book these criteria elements have not been developed in detail.	

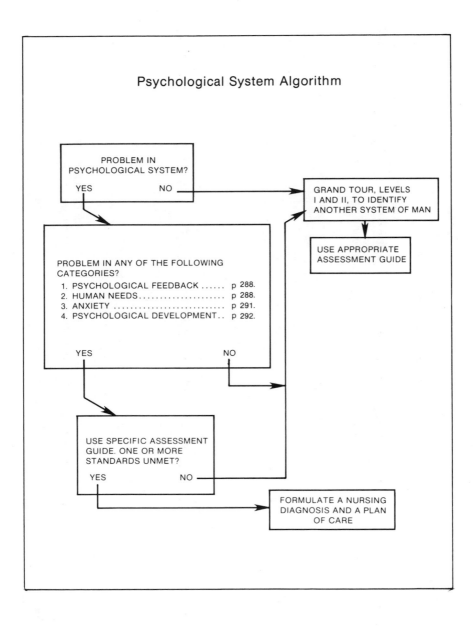

Psychological System Algorithm

PROBLEM IN
PSYCHOLOGICAL SYSTEM?

YES   NO

GRAND TOUR, LEVELS
I AND II, TO IDENTIFY
ANOTHER SYSTEM OF MAN

USE APPROPRIATE
ASSESSMENT GUIDE

PROBLEM IN ANY OF THE FOLLOWING
CATEGORIES?
1. PSYCHOLOGICAL FEEDBACK ...... p 288.
2. HUMAN NEEDS..................... p 288.
3. ANXIETY .... p 291.
4. PSYCHOLOGICAL DEVELOPMENT.. p 292.

YES   NO

USE SPECIFIC ASSESSMENT
GUIDE. ONE OR MORE
STANDARDS UNMET?

YES   NO

FORMULATE A NURSING
DIAGNOSIS AND A PLAN
OF CARE

Psychological System
1. Psychological Feedback

CRITERIA	HEALTH STANDARDS	METHODS OF MEASUREMENT QUESTIONS, OBSERVATIONS, INSPECTIONS
Systems Theory: Bertalanffy[1] — Psychological phenomena such as creativity and self-realization are parts of man's feedback system.		
Creativity[15,24] Questioning Accountability Flexibility Curiosity	Evidence of capacity to extend self-experience and awareness and seek own potential.	For the purposes of this book, specific methods of measurement derived from systems and needs/motivation theory have not been formulated.
Self-realization Synthesis Evaluation	Ability to develop conceptual relationships, to predict outcomes, produce plans, evaluate effectiveness of actions.	

Psychological System
2. Human Needs

CRITERIA	HEALTH STANDARDS	METHODS OF MEASUREMENT QUESTIONS, OBSERVATIONS, INSPECTIONS
Need/Motivation Theories: Maslow, A. — Maslow's hierarchy identifies psychological levels of human needs and safety; love; esteem; and self-actualization.[18]		

Emotional needs

Security   Perceived sense of emotional
                            security.

Affection   Perceived feelings of affec-
                            tion and belonging by and
                            toward significant others.

Recognition   Perceived sense of recogni-
                            tion for accomplishments.

Self-determination   Perceived satisfaction relative
                            to achievement of own potential.

Fried, E. — "One of the most basic human needs is activeness...drive towards assertiveness, stimulation and
exploration."[25]

Activeness   Ability to assert one's will
                            and skills in new situations
                            and in human contacts.

Assertiveness   Ability to feel strong
                            emotions.

Stimulation   Ability to make choices
                            and initiate action.

Exploration   Presence of feelings and
                            curiosity and stimulation.

                            No evidence of passivity,
                            conformity and regression.

2. Human Needs (cont.)

CRITERIA	HEALTH STANDARDS	METHODS OF MEASUREMENT QUESTIONS, OBSERVATIONS, INSPECTIONS
Rogers, C. — An individual is basically guided by needs for growth and self-actualization.[26]		
Growth	Presence of feelings of security, positive self-esteem and trust in one's own feelings and perceptions.	
Self-actualization		
Buhler, C. — Man is motivated by basic intrinsic needs: pleasure; fitting-in; creative expansion; ordering of events.[27]		
Intrinsic needs	Perceived balance between assertiveness and conformity.	
Pleasure	Perceived feelings of satisfaction with sexuality, love, and ego recognition.	
Fitting-in	Perceived feelings of belonging.	
Creative expansion	Evidence of self-expression and creative accomplishments.	
Ordering of events	Evidence of past and present ability to structure life.	

Psychological System

3. Anxiety

CRITERIA	HEALTH STANDARDS	METHODS OF MEASUREMENT QUESTIONS, OBSERVATIONS, INSPECTIONS
Peplau, H. — A certain level of anxiety is necessary to initiate activity. Anxiety occurs in degrees forming a continuum from mild anxiety to panic.[28]		
Levels of anxiety	Being alert, consciously aware of stimuli and perceptive, with associated behavior changes.	For the purposes of this book, specific methods of measurement derived from Peplau's theory of anxiety have not been formulated.
Mild	Evidence of independent problem-solving activity.	
Moderate	Ability to problem-solve with help. Presence of decreased perception, selective concentration, decreased learning.	
Severe Panic	No evidence of:	
	Decreased perceptions	
	Decreased attention span	
	Scattered attention	
	Physical and emotional discomfort	
	Dread and sorrow	
	Automatic relief behavior (flight somatization)	
	Disoriented perception	

Psychological System

4. Psychological Development

CRITERIA	HEALTH STANDARDS	METHODS OF MEASUREMENT QUESTIONS, OBSERVATIONS, INSPECTIONS
Growth and Development: Erickson, E. — There are eight phases of psychological development that occur at predictable periods throughout life.[29]		
Psychological development	Progressive accomplishment of psychological tasks by the maximum age of each phase.	For the purposes of this book, specific methods of measurement for Erickson's theory of growth and development have not been formulated.
	Evidence of:	
Trust versus mistrust (birth — 1 year)	Trust at least in relationship with mother — birth to 1 yr.	
Autonomy versus shame, doubt (2-4 years)	Assertiveness of child's own will.	
Initiative versus guilt (4-5 years)	Social contacts outside of family.	
Industry versus inferiority (6-11 years)	Ability to differentiate between work and play, understanding expectations and peers.	
Identity versus identity diffusion (12 to 18 years)	Ability to identify own preferences. Ability to evaluate own sexuality.	

Intimacy and solidarity versus isolation (young adulthood)	Sexuality, love relationships, leadership roles and personal assertiveness
Generativity versus stagnation (middle years)	Focus on guiding the next generation.
Integrity versus despair (old age)	Increasing consistency of personality traits with one's own underlying needs and desires.[30]
	Positive feelings toward aging.[31]
	Redefining and adjusting physical and social space.[31]
	Perceived feelings of pride and usefulness.[31]
	Striving toward personal goals.[31]

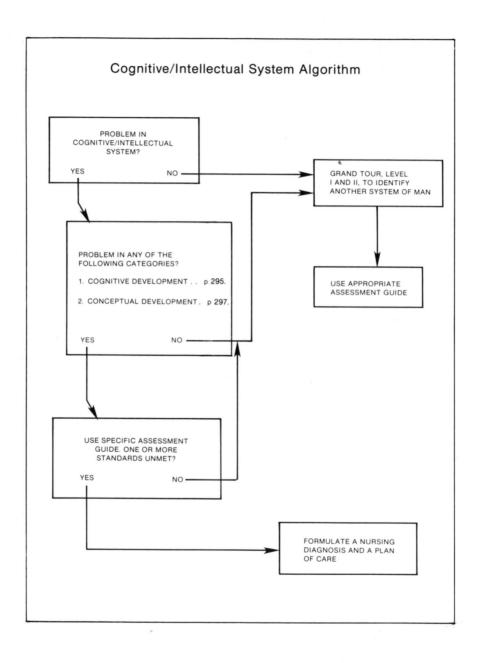

Cognitive/Intellectual System Algorithm

PROBLEM IN
COGNITIVE/INTELLECTUAL
SYSTEM?

YES   NO

GRAND TOUR, LEVEL
I AND II, TO IDENTIFY
ANOTHER SYSTEM OF MAN

PROBLEM IN ANY OF THE
FOLLOWING CATEGORIES?

1. COGNITIVE DEVELOPMENT . . p 295.

2. CONCEPTUAL DEVELOPMENT . p 297.

YES   NO

USE APPROPRIATE
ASSESSMENT GUIDE

USE SPECIFIC ASSESSMENT
GUIDE. ONE OR MORE
STANDARDS UNMET?

YES   NO

FORMULATE A NURSING
DIAGNOSIS AND A PLAN
OF CARE

Cognitive/Intellectual System
1. Cognitive Development

CRITERIA	HEALTH STANDARDS	METHODS OF MEASUREMENT QUESTIONS, OBSERVATIONS, INSPECTIONS
Piaget, J. — Cognitive development is an active process, resulting in an individual's ability to absorb increasingly complex experiences. There are four sequential developmental stages from birth to early adolescence.[32]		
Cognitive development	Progressive accomplishment of cognitive developmental tasks by the maximum age of each stage.	For the purposes of this book, specific methods of measurement for cognitive and learning theories have not been formulated.
Stage One (birth - 2 years)	Evidence of coordinating action with perceptions.	
	Ability to follow object with eyes.	
	Evidence of experimentation and exploration.	
Stage Two (2-7 years)	Evidence of experimentation with language.	
	Ability to manipulate objects in environment.	
	Participation in imaginative play.	
	Evidence of questioning and talking.	

1. Cognitive Development *(cont.)*

Stage Three (7-11 years)

Evidence of listening and experimenting.

Ability to organize facts about real world.

Selective use of facts for problem-solving.

Performing concrete operations.

Ability to reason inductively.

Knowledge of spatial relationships, matter, weight, length and volume.

Stage Four (12-15 years)

Ability to reason hypothetically, deductively and logically.

Belbin, E. and Belbin, R. — An adult's intellectual development is characterized by three major cognitive skills: controller performance; memorized skills; understanding limited by overly complex or overly simple situations.[33]

Controlled performance

Ability to perform under conditions of speed, stress and difficulty.

Memorized skills

Ability to identify previously incorrect behavior or responses.[34,35,36]

Understanding

Ability to recognize overly complex or overly simple situations.

	The ability to recall and use skills in the face of distraction.

Neugarten, B. and Birren, J.[38] — As a person ages, one need not expect deterioration of mental functioning. There are heightened executive processes which are designed to meet one's own ends.

Executive processes	Sustained executive processes throughout the adult life span.
	Evidence of (in the absence of poor health):
	Self-awareness
	Selectivity
	Manipulation and control of environment
	Mastery
	Competence in a wide array of cognitive strategies
	Control over impulses

Cognitive/Intellectual System
2. Conceptual Relationships

CRITERIA	HEALTH STANDARDS	METHODS OF MEASUREMENT QUESTIONS, OBSERVATIONS, INSPECTIONS

Lewin, K. — Learning is a matter of understanding relationships within a total field or area.[39]

| Conceptual relationships | Ability to draw relationships within a given context. | |

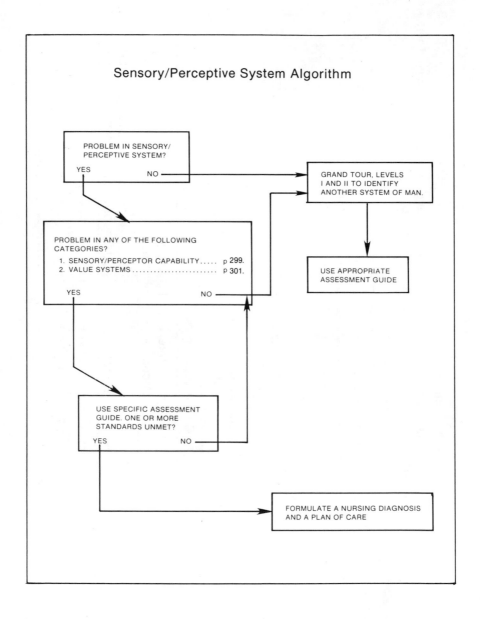

Sensory/Perceptive System Algorithm

PROBLEM IN SENSORY/
PERCEPTIVE SYSTEM?

YES   NO

GRAND TOUR, LEVELS
I AND II TO IDENTIFY
ANOTHER SYSTEM OF MAN.

PROBLEM IN ANY OF THE FOLLOWING
CATEGORIES?
1. SENSORY/PERCEPTOR CAPABILITY..... p 299.
2. VALUE SYSTEMS .... p 301.

YES   NO

USE APPROPRIATE
ASSESSMENT GUIDE

USE SPECIFIC ASSESSMENT
GUIDE. ONE OR MORE
STANDARDS UNMET?

YES   NO

FORMULATE A NURSING DIAGNOSIS
AND A PLAN OF CARE

Sensory/Perceptive System
1. Sensory Receptor Capability

Rose, A.[40] and Day, R.[41] — Perception is the ability to place values and create symbols. For perception, there must be receptor capability; transformation and energy coding; and recall, labeling or predicting.

CRITERIA	HEALTH STANDARDS	METHODS OF MEASUREMENT QUESTIONS, OBSERVATIONS, INSPECTIONS
Basic orienting systems: Touch Sight Hearing Taste and smell	Presence of intact sensory receptors.	Assess according to physiological system of man, algorithm 17.
Transforming and energy coding	Ability to recall consequential facts or events.	
Central neural storage.	Selective responses to stimuli that are consistent with the environment and organism itself.	Has anything like this happened to you before? If yes, how did you respond the last time? How is the situation similar or different to what happened before? Do you know anyone else that this has happened to?
Peripheral neural activity.	Selective responses to stimuli that are consistent with the environment and organism itself.	Inspect according to physiological system of man: neurological testing for pressure, temperature, pain, light, taste, smell, spatial relations, sound and orientation to time,

1. Sensory Receptor Capability *(cont.)*

CRITERIA	HEALTH STANDARDS	METHODS OF MEASUREMENT QUESTIONS, OBSERVATIONS, INSPECTIONS
		Algorithms 11, 13 and 17.
		Observe for blocking and interrupted train of thought, meaningless repetition or echoing of words.

Central neural activity
  Organizing
  Labeling
	Ability to organize and label events, objects, and situations.	What do these symptoms or the situation mean to you?
		Perform object-naming test.

Predicting	Ability to predict consequences of a situation based on previous and current perceptions.	How do you feel about what is happening to you? How does your family feel about what is happening to you or this situation? What choices or alternatives seem available right now?
		How is each alternative likely to work out?
		Observe ease and rate with which questions are answered and coherence and continuity of speech.

Sensory/Perceptive System
2. Value Systems

CRITERIA	HEALTH STANDARDS	METHODS OF MEASUREMENT QUESTIONS, OBSERVATIONS, INSPECTIONS
Perception Theory: Vernon — Perception determines how one behaves. Perceptions are influenced by value systems and experiences.[42]		
Perception	Behavior consistent with own values.	How easy or difficult is it for you to participate in this situation right now?
		How do you feel about yourself right now?
Values Meanings Meanings Symbols		Observe for: Muscular tension Distracted or random movements Anxious facial expressions Disturbances of thought process Tone of voice
Growth and Development: Dieklemann, N.[43] and Sheehy, G.[44] — In adulthood, man questions himself and his values. Life structures and values are shed and rebuilt every seven years.		
Questioning of values	Evidence of periodic questioning one's self and one's values in adulthood with associated behavior change.	For the purposes of this book, specific methods of measurement derived from theories of growth and development and cognitive dissonance have not been formulated.
Self in relationship to others.		
Safeness or danger.		

2. Value Systems (cont.)

CRITERIA	HEALTH STANDARDS	METHODS OF MEASUREMENT QUESTIONS, OBSERVATIONS, INSPECTIONS
Aliveness or stagnation.		
Stress: Festinger, L. — Theory of Cognitive Dissonance: Perceived stress creates dissonance and results in tension-reducing behaviors.[45]		
Perceived stress	Evidence of tension-reducing behavior resulting in a feeling of comfort.	
Dissonance		
Tension reduction		

Interactive/Affiliative System
1. Interpersonal Relationships

CRITERIA	HEALTH STANDARDS	METHODS OF MEASUREMENT QUESTIONS, OBSERVATIONS, INSPECTIONS
Interpersonal Theory: Sullivan — Tension reduction and security combine to become the major behavior goals of any individual. These goals require feelings of approval and prestige. A person's self-concept or self-dynamism organizes behavior and is a result of past and present experiences with significant others. Behavior, emotions and needs originate from the interaction of one individual with another. Anxiety is the chief disruptive force in interpersonal relationships. Interpersonal security is a major human need. Past relationships influence perceptions of present relationships. In-security in interpersonal relationships produces anxiety. A person will interact or not interact to reduce anxiety. Present interactions are influenced by perceptions of past interactions.[46,47,48]		
Interpersonal security	Presence of feelings of security in most important interpersonal relationships.	How do you feel about what is happening to you?
Feelings of approval		Put down

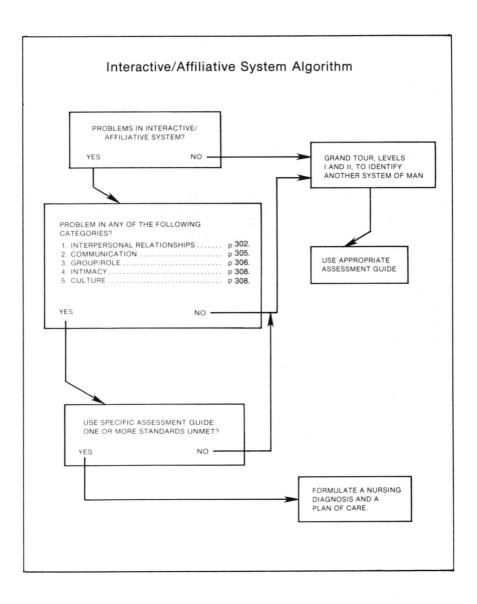

Interactive/Affiliative System Algorithm

PROBLEMS IN INTERACTIVE/
AFFILIATIVE SYSTEM?

YES   NO

GRAND TOUR, LEVELS
I AND II, TO IDENTIFY
ANOTHER SYSTEM OF MAN

PROBLEM IN ANY OF THE FOLLOWING
CATEGORIES?
1. INTERPERSONAL RELATIONSHIPS . . . . p 302.
2. COMMUNICATION . . . . p 305.
3. GROUP/ROLE . . . . p 306.
4. INTIMACY . . . . p 308.
5. CULTURE . . . . p 308.

YES   NO

USE APPROPRIATE
ASSESSMENT GUIDE

USE SPECIFIC ASSESSMENT GUIDE.
ONE OR MORE STANDARDS UNMET?

YES   NO

FORMULATE A NURSING
DIAGNOSIS AND A
PLAN OF CARE.

1. Interpersonal Relationships *(cont.)*

CRITERIA	HEALTH STANDARDS	METHODS OF MEASUREMENT QUESTIONS, OBSERVATIONS, INSPECTIONS
Feelings of prestige Symptoms of anxiety Self-dynamism		Not valued or recognized Do you feel you have control over what is happening to you? Has something like this ever happened before? What do you remember about it? Who, if anyone, can help you (be supportive to you) at this time? Who are the most important people in your life? Family Significant others Work group Social group Do these relationships with these people make you feel comfortable/uncomfortable? Now Past Potential in future What interactions, if any, tend to upset you? Observe body language Posture

Muscle tension
Facial expressions
Random/compulsive movements
Tone of voice

Interactive/Affiliative System
2. Communication

CRITERIA	HEALTH STANDARDS	METHODS OF MEASUREMENT QUESTIONS, OBSERVATIONS, INSPECTIONS
Communication Theory: Reusch — Communication results when one mind is able to affect another. Transmitting, receiving, and validating are necessary for communication.[49]		
Communication Behavior change Information processing	Ability to at least change the behavior of self or others in an attempt to reduce uncertainty in the most important life situations.	How do you usually find out what others expect of you? How easy or difficult is it for you to follow through? In your past, how have you been able to respond to your own or others' expectations. Do you usually feel in control of the situation or a victim of the circumstances?
Bevis[50] — Human productivity and survival are dependent upon communication — interpersonal, intrapersonal and community.		

2. Communication (cont.)

CRITERIA	HEALTH STANDARDS	METHODS OF MEASUREMENT QUESTIONS, OBSERVATIONS, INSPECTIONS
Productivity Survival	Ability to communicate well enough to survive according to one's own definition.	How have you generally responded to pressures for change in your life? What type of work do you do? How do you spend your leisure time? How do you feel about your achievements in life? What important things do you feel you have accomplished? Observe for: Transmitting ideas Receiving or understanding Validating or checking out

Interactive/Affiliative System
3. Group/Role

CRITERIA	HEALTH STANDARDS	METHODS OF MEASUREMENT QUESTIONS, OBSERVATIONS, INSPECTIONS
Roles	A state of being that is con-	Is there someone/s on whom you rely?

Robbins — How a person behaves is determined by the role defined in a given context. When a group exists, role perceptions and expectations exist. Role conflict occurs when one or more group/s' expectations cannot be met. Lost roles lead to identity problems. Lost roles, if replaced, minimize identity crisis.[51]

Social kin networks	sistent with the values and norms of the most important reference groups.	How easy is it to keep in touch with those who are important to you?
		What groups are you affiliated with?
	Evidence of membership in a social group.	Which do you feel most comfortable with?
	Evidence of a place in a kin network.	How consistent are your opinions and feelings with those in the group?
	Perceived sense of comfort with values and norms of reference groups.	Which groups are the most important to you?
		How able are you to meet their expectations?
Loyalties	Ability to rank loyalties among reference groups.	Which roles do you assume right now in your life?
Perceived roles	Satisfaction with role identity.	Which role is most important?
		Are you satisfied with this role?
		Observe body language
		Posture
		Muscle tension
		Facial expressions
		Random/compulsive movements
		Tone of voice

Interactive/Affiliative System
4. Intimacy

CRITERIA	HEALTH STANDARDS	METHODS OF MEASUREMENT QUESTIONS, OBSERVATIONS, INSPECTIONS
Intimacy Theory: Angyal — The maintenance of closeness with another is the center of existence up to the very end of life.[52]		
Intimacy	Closeness with another throughout life.	What about close personal relationships in your life?

Interactive/Affiliative System
5. Culture

CRITERIA	HEALTH STANDARDS	METHODS OF MEASUREMENT QUESTIONS, OBSERVATIONS, INSPECTIONS
Culture Theory: Robbins,[51] Mead,[53] and Sumner[54] — Man's wishes, needs, desires, value system and behavior norms are determined by reference groups.		
Values, behaviors and goals	State of being that is consistent with the values, norms and goals of the most important reference groups.	Assess according to Group/Role, Algorithm Three.

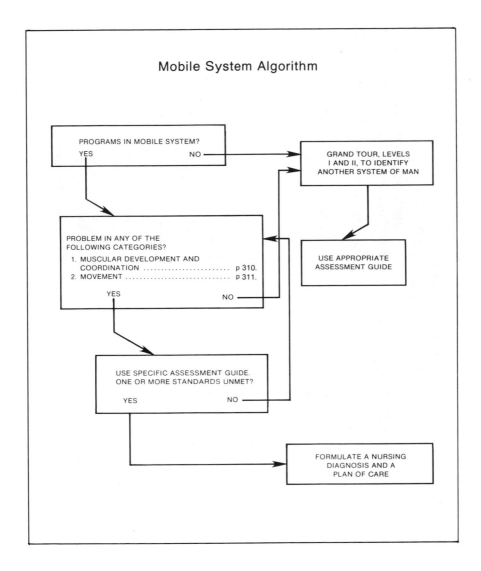

Mobile System Algorithm

PROGRAMS IN MOBILE SYSTEM?
YES   NO

GRAND TOUR, LEVELS
I AND II, TO IDENTIFY
ANOTHER SYSTEM OF MAN

PROBLEM IN ANY OF THE
FOLLOWING CATEGORIES?
1. MUSCULAR DEVELOPMENT AND
   COORDINATION .... p 310.
2. MOVEMENT .... p 311.
   YES   NO

USE APPROPRIATE
ASSESSMENT GUIDE

USE SPECIFIC ASSESSMENT GUIDE.
ONE OR MORE STANDARDS UNMET?
   YES   NO

FORMULATE A NURSING
DIAGNOSIS AND A
PLAN OF CARE

Mobile System of Man
1. Muscular Development and Coordination

CRITERIA	HEALTH STANDARDS	METHODS OF MEASUREMENT QUESTIONS, OBSERVATIONS, INSPECTIONS
Mobility Theory: Barsch, R. — Movement is one of three critical capabilities for man's survival.[55]		
Mobility	Presence of muscular development and motor coordination consistent with age allowing for free and safe movement.	Assess according to Physiological System of man, Algorithms 12 and 13.
Muscular development		
Muscular coordination		
Space	Adequate space in which to exercise movement and to express self through gestures, mannerisms and leisure activities.	Observe for presence of:
		Obstacles to movement.
		Policies that enhance or limit movement.
		Stimuli; i.e., color, patterns.
		Social norms that affect movement.
		Transport systems; i.e., wheelchairs, crutches, subway.
		Are you able to move about enough to accomplish those things you need to do?
		Are you able to move about enough to accomplish those things you like to do?
		How do you express your feelings through movement?

Mobile System
2. Movement

CRITERIA	HEALTH STANDARDS	METHODS OF MEASUREMENT QUESTIONS, OBSERVATIONS, INSPECTIONS
Systems Theory: For man to interact with his environment in a dynamic continuous interchange, five elements of mobility are essential: dynamic balance, feedback creating a body image; spatial awareness; time related to action or activity; biological, habit and environmental rhythms.[55]		
	Ability to:	For the purposes of this book, specific methods of measurement derived from systems theory and culture theory have not been formulated.
Movement	Move within range of growth and development.	
Body image	Describe perception of own body.	
Spatial relations	Estimate, organize, and measure space consistent with developmental age.	
Time awareness	Estimate required time to complete action or activity.	
Biological rhythms	Identify timing of activities of daily living: cycles of energy, sleep, hunger, temperature, evacuation.	
Environmental constraints	Predict uncontrollable environmental constraints that dictate timing: work	

2. Movement (cont.)

CRITERIA	HEALTH STANDARDS	METHODS OF MEASUREMENT QUESTIONS, OBSERVATIONS, INSPECTIONS
	schedules, seasonal changes, temperature, demands of others, etc.	
Culture Theory: Mead, M. —	Cultural values determine the mode and frequency of mobility.[53]	
Transportation systems	Ability to use accessible transportation systems.	

REFERENCES

1. Bertalanffy L Von: *General System Theory.* New York, Brazillar, 1968, p 193.
2. Buckley W: *Sociology and Modern Systems Theory.* Englewood Cliffs, NJ, Prentice Hall, 1967.
3. Koestler A: *The Ghost in the Machine.* New York, MacMillan, 1967, p 47.
4. Boulding K: General Systems Theory — The Skeleton of Science. In Buckley W (ed): *Modern System Research for The Behavior Scientist.* Englewood Cliffs, NJ, Prentice-Hall, 1968, pp 3-10.
5. Beland I, Passos J: *Clinical Nursing, Pathophysiological and Psychosocial Approaches.* 3rd ed, New York, MacMillan Publishing Co, Inc, 1975, pp 58, 61, 63, 68, 872.
6. Davidson I, Henry J: *Total Sanford Clinical Diagnoses by Laboratory Methods.* 4th ed, Philadelphia, WB Saunders and Co, 1969.
7. Beyers M, Dudas S: *The Clinical Practice of Medical-Surgical Nursing.* Boston, Little-Brown and Co, 1977, p 15.
8. Rogers M: *Theoretical Basis of Nursing.* Philadelphia, FA Davis Co, 1970, p 97.
9. Dunn H: High level wellness means for man and society. American Jnl Pub Health 49:788, June 1959.
10. Bates B: *A Guide to Physical Examination.* Philadelphia, JB Lippincott Co, 1974, pp 46-47, 81-115, 166, 228-237.
11. Shafer K et al: *Medical-Surgical Nursing.* 6th ed, St Louis, CV Mosby Co, 1975, p 97.
12. Gillies D, Alyn I: *Patient Assessment and Management by the Nurse Practitioner.* Philadelphia, WB Saunders Co, 1976, pp 29-31, 51-53, 93, 222.
13. Selye H: *The Stress of Life.* New York, McGraw Hill, 1956.
14. Selye H: *The Stress Syndrome. Am J Nurs,* March 1965.
15. Sutterly D, Donnally G: *Perspectives in Human Development — Nursing Throughout the Life Cycle.* Philadelphia, JB Lippincott Co, 1973, pp 180-182, 208.
16. Luckman J, Sorensen K: *Medical-Surgical Nursing, A Psychophysiological Approach.* Philadelphia, WB Saunders Co, 1974, pp 112-114.
17. Bordicks K: *Patterns of Shock, Implications for Nursing Care.* New York, Macmillan Co, 1965.
18. Maslow A: *Motivation and Personality.* 2nd ed, New York, Harper and Row, 1970.
19. Murray M: *Fundamentals of Nursing.* Englewood Cliffs, NJ, Prentice Hall Inc, 1976, p 339-390.
20. Sana J, Judge R: *Physical Appraisal Methods in Nursing Practice.* Boston, Little Brown and Co, 1975, pp 171-206, 259-274.
21. Gartland J: *Fundamentals of Orthopedics.* 2nd ed, Philadelphia, WB Saunders Co, 1974, p 9.
22. Sherman J, Fields S: *Guide to Patient Evaluation.* Flushing, NY, Medical Examination Publishing Co, Inc, 1974, pp 101-120.
23. Tanner J, Taylor G (eds): Growth. Time-Life Science Books, New York, Time Inc, 1965, p 9.
24. Fromm E: The Creative Attitude. In Anderson H (ed): *Creativity and its Cultivation.* New York, Harper & Bros., 1959, pp 44-54.
25. Fried E: *Active/Passive: The Crucial Psychological Dimension.* New York, Greene and Statton, 1970, p 3.
26. Rogers C: *Client-Centered Therapy.* Boston, Houghton-Mifflin Co, 1951.
27. Buhler C: Basic theoretical concepts of humanistic psychology. *Amer Psychol* 26:4:378-386, 1971.
28. Peplau H: A Working Definition of Anxiety in *Some Clinical Approaches to Psychiatric Nursing.* Burd S, Marshall M (eds): New York, MacMillan Co, 1963, pp 323-327.
29. Erickson E: *Childhood and Society.* 2nd ed, New York, WW Norton, 1963.
30. Neugarten B, Havighurst R, Tobin S: Personality and Patterns of Aging. In Neugarten,

B (ed): *Middle Age and Aging.* Chicago, University of Chicago Press, 1968, pp 173-177.
31. Lewis M, Butler R: Life review therapy — putting memories to work in individual and group psychotherapy. *Geriatrics* 165-173, November 1974.
32. Piaget J: *Genetic Epistemology.* New York, WW Norton and Co, Inc, 1964.
33. Belbin E, Belbin R: New Careers in Middle Age. In *Proceedings of Seventh International Congress of Gerontology.* Vienna, 1966.
34. Skinner B: *Science and Human Behavior.* New York, Macmillan Co, 1953.
35. Bigge M: *Learning Theories for Teachers.* New York, Harper and Row Publishers, 1971.
36. Gagne R: *The Conditions of Learning.* New York, Holt, Rinehart and Winston Inc, 1965.
37. Neugarten B: The Awareness of Middle Age. In Neugarten B (ed): *Middle Age and Aging.* Chicago, The University of Chicago Press, 1968, pp 93-98.
38. Birren J: Psychological aspects of aging: intellectual functioning. *Gerontologist* 8:16-19, 1968.
39. Lewin K: Fixed Theory and Learning. In Henry N (ed): *The Forty-First Yearbook for the Study of Education, Part Two: The Psychology of Learning.* Chicago, The University of Chicago Press, 1942, pp 215-245.
40. Rose A: A Systematic Summary of Symbolic Interaction Theory. In Riehl J, Roy S (eds): *Conceptual Models in Nursing.* New York, Appleton-Century-Crofts, 1974, p 35.
41. Day R: *Perception.* Dubuque, Iowa, Wm C Brown Co, 1966, pp 6-9, 42-43.
42. Vernon M: *Perception Through Experience.* London, England, Methuen and Co, Ltd, 1970, pp 1-240.
43. Dieklemann N: *Primary Health Care of the Well Adult.* New York, McGraw-Hill Book Co, 1977, pp 9-12.
44. Sheehy G: Passages: *Predictable Crises of Adult Life.* New York, EP Dutton and Co, Inc 1976.
45. Festinger L: *A Theory of Cognitive Dissonance.* Standord, Calif, Stanford, University Press, 1957.
46. Sullivan H: *Conceptions of Modern Psychiatry.* Washington, DC, Wm Alason White Psychiatric Foundation, 1947, p 142, 119-174.
47. Sullivan H: *The Interpersonal Theory of Psychiatry.* New York, WW Norton and Co, Inc, 1953.
48. Sullivan H: Introduction to the study of interpersonal relations. *J Psychiatr* 1:121-134, 1938.
49. Reusch J: General theory of communication. In Arieti S (ed): *Amer Handbood of Psychiatry,* New York, WW Norton and Co, Inc, 1961.
50. Bevis E: *Curriculum Building in Nursing, A Process.* St. Louis, CV Mosby Co, 1973, p 75.
51. Robbins S: *The Administrative Process, Integrating Theory and Practice.* Englewood Cliffs, NJ, Prentice-Hall Inc, 1976, pp 283-284.
52. Angyal A: *Neurosis and Treatment, A Holistic Theory.* New York, John Wiley and Sons, 1965.
53. Mead M (ed): *Cultural Patterns and Technical Change.* UNESCO, New York, A Mentor Book, pp 12-13.
54. Sumner W: *Folkways.* New York, Ginn, 1906, pp 12-13.
55. Barsch R: *Achieving Perceptual Motor Efficiency: A Space Oriented Approach to Learning.* Vol I, Seattle, Wash, Special Child Publications, 1967.

APPENDIX B
Assessment Guides:
Theories of Man
and Environment

**APPENDIX B
ASSESSMENT GUIDES:
THEORIES OF MAN AND ENVIRONMENT**

Appendix B is a compilation of assessment guides. It is divided into five sections corresponding with the five systems of man's environment: economic, physical, mobile, demographic, and social/cultural. Each section is preceded by an algorithm flow chart. The flow chart assumes that first and second grand-tour questions have been asked and that a speculation has been made as to which system or systems of man's environment are likely problem areas. The flow chart uses Yes-No decision choices at several junctures, leading one either through a detailed assessment pathway (resulting in a nursing diagnosis), or through a pathway that bypasses detailed assessments leading one to another system of man or environment.

The assessment questions, observations, and examinations are designed to gather information about man as he is affected by his environment. No attempt has been made to design detailed assessment guides for the environment as it is affected by man. Although reciprocal adaptation is one of the guiding theories of the conceptual framework, the development of assessment guides are here limited to the effects of the environment upon man. Screening questions only have been developed for the environment assessment perspective; they can be found in Chapter 4, Table 4.2.

Also for the purposes of this text, several assessment guides are not developed in complete detail. The intent is to illustrate a process which may be used by experts in a given area of nursing to formulate their own in-depth assessment algorithms. Some of the systems of the environment include no assessment questions, observations, and examinations; however, summaries of theories, criteria, and health standards are completely detailed. As with the systems of man, the authors have used their own best judgment in summarizing theories, extracting criteria, and formulating standards and methods of measurement.

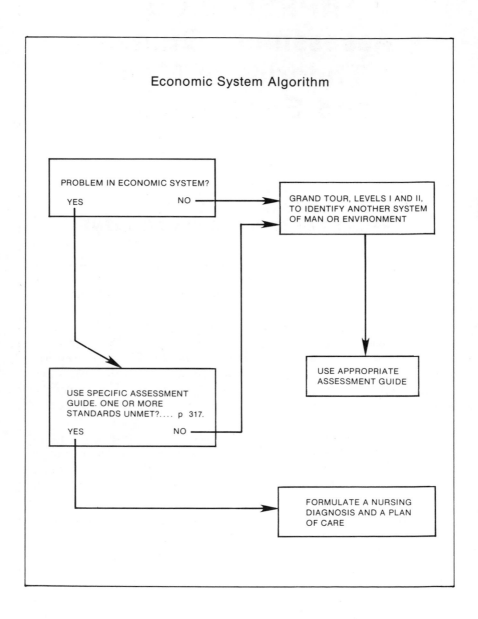

Economic System Algorithm

PROBLEM IN ECONOMIC SYSTEM?

YES   NO

GRAND TOUR, LEVELS I AND II, TO IDENTIFY ANOTHER SYSTEM OF MAN OR ENVIRONMENT

USE SPECIFIC ASSESSMENT GUIDE. ONE OR MORE STANDARDS UNMET?.... p 317.

YES   NO

USE APPROPRIATE ASSESSMENT GUIDE

FORMULATE A NURSING DIAGNOSIS AND A PLAN OF CARE

Economic System

CRITERIA	HEALTH STANDARDS	METHODS OF MEASUREMENT QUESTIONS, OBSERVATIONS, INSPECTIONS
Systems: Spencer[1,2] — The economic system involves input (labor, land, capital), processes (technology, specialization, and exchange systems), and outputs (standards of living).		
Economic system	Condition of supply and demand which allows the system to achieve the desired standard of living.	For the purposes of this book, specific methods of measurement derived from systems and supply and demand theories have not been formulated.
Input	Evidence of labor, land, and capital.	
Process	Utilization of technology, specialization, and exchange.	
Output	Presence of a definable standard of living.	
Theory of Supply and Demand:[1,3] Supply is the amount of goods or services which producers are willing to sell. Demand is the amount of goods or services consumers will buy. Elasticity, inelasticity, and contrived demand are elements of the supply-and-demand theory.		
Supply and demand	Reasonable availability of goods and services.	
	Purchasing power for goods and services.	
	Flexibility of desire versus need.	

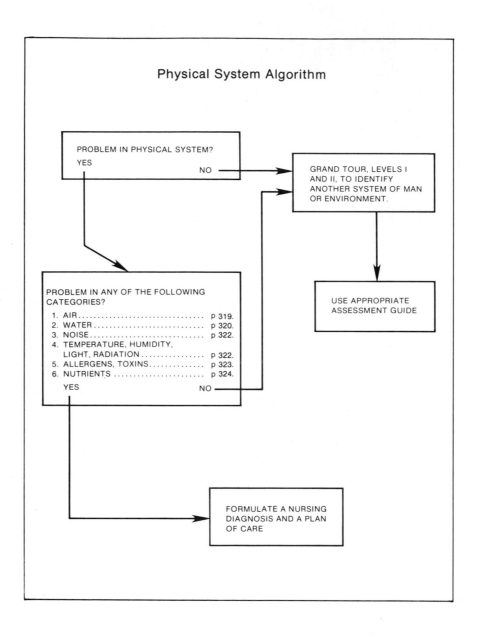

Physical System Algorithm

PROBLEM IN PHYSICAL SYSTEM?

YES

NO

GRAND TOUR, LEVELS I AND II, TO IDENTIFY ANOTHER SYSTEM OF MAN OR ENVIRONMENT.

PROBLEM IN ANY OF THE FOLLOWING CATEGORIES?

1. AIR................................. p 319.
2. WATER............................. p 320.
3. NOISE.............................. p 322.
4. TEMPERATURE, HUMIDITY, LIGHT, RADIATION................ p 322.
5. ALLERGENS, TOXINS.............. p 323.
6. NUTRIENTS .... p 324.

YES

NO

USE APPROPRIATE ASSESSMENT GUIDE

FORMULATE A NURSING DIAGNOSIS AND A PLAN OF CARE

Physical System
1. Air

Systems: All organisms modify their environment and are modified by it. These interactions are known as ecological systems. The physical system is comprised of air; water; noise; temperature; humidity and light; radiation; allergens; toxins; nutrients; and other hazards.[4]

CRITERIA	HEALTH STANDARDS	METHODS OF MEASUREMENT QUESTIONS, OBSERVATIONS, INSPECTIONS
Physical elements		
Air[5]	A state of air containing 20% oxygen and a composition of air containing no more than the minimum safe standards of pollution.	Inspect for any special environmental situations that may create oxygen content lesser or greater than ambiant air (hyperbaric chamber; isolette; inhalation equipment; crowded therapy rooms, unventilated rooms).
	Sulfur oxide, less than 80μ Mgm/m³ annual mean.	Do you live, work or spend most of your time in places where you are exposed to:
	Nitrogen oxide, less than 0.05 ppm annual mean.	Industrial fumes? Heavy traffic? Smoke, soot? Refineries?
	Particulates, 75μ Mgm/m³ annual mean.	
	Hydrocarbons, 0.24 ppm in 3-hour concentrations once per year.	Obtain pollution data.

1. Air (cont.)

CRITERIA	HEALTH STANDARDS	METHODS OF MEASUREMENT QUESTIONS, OBSERVATIONS, INSPECTIONS
	Carbon monoxide, 9 ppm in 8-hour concentrations once per year.	
	Photochemical oxidants, 0.08 ppm maximum/hour concentration each year.	Is the climate normally sunny where you live?
	Tar not to exceed 9 ppm. 1 puff of cigarette = 600 ppm.	Do you smoke or are you exposed to someone who does smoke?

Physical System
2. Water

CRITERIA	HEALTH STANDARDS	METHODS OF MEASUREMENT QUESTIONS, OBSERVATIONS, INSPECTIONS
Water[5]	Potable water according to state standards.	Inspect type of water supply. Secure and visually inspect a sample of water.
	Composition of water not to exceed maximum contaminant levels.	Do you receive your water from a public water supply?

CRITERIA	HEALTH STANDARDS	METHODS OF MEASUREMENT QUESTIONS, OBSERVATIONS, INSPECTIONS
Choliform bacteria Extraneous matter, inorganic matter		If not, how does your water taste, smell, and appear? Do you or your family have episodes of nausea, vomiting or diarrhea? Where is your water supply in relation to waste effluents?

Physical System
3. Noise

CRITERIA	HEALTH STANDARDS	METHODS OF MEASUREMENT QUESTIONS, OBSERVATIONS, INSPECTIONS
Noise[5]	Sound levels not to exceed 120 decibels. Environment free of high frequency sound. Environment free from potential sudden, severe noise or chronic long-term noise.	Do you live or work in places where there are any of the following kinds of noises: High frequency, shrill, sudden, severe, constant, disruptive? Idling buses? Food blenders? Subway trains? Noisy kitchens? Outboard motors? Car racing? Power motors? Motorcycles? Rock music with amplifiers? Pneumatic riveters?

3. Noise *(cont.)*

CRITERIA	HEALTH STANDARDS	METHODS OF MEASUREMENT QUESTIONS, OBSERVATIONS, INSPECTIONS
		Power saws?
		Jet roar?
		Rocket engines?
		In the presence of any of these factors, when was your last hearing test?
		Is there any particular noise that you find bothersome?
		Have you noticed any change in your hearing?

Physical System

4. Temperature, Humidity, Light, Radiation

CRITERIA	HEALTH STANDARDS	METHODS OF MEASUREMENT QUESTIONS, OBSERVATIONS, INSPECTIONS
Temperature	Temperature within comfort range.	Does the temperature of your environment feel comfortable?
Humidity	Humidity within comfort range.	Is the air either too moist, too dry, or comfortable?

		METHODS OF MEASUREMENT QUESTIONS, OBSERVATIONS, INSPECTIONS
Light	Light available to accomplish necessary activities.	Do you have enough light to see easily and to enable you to perform necessary tasks? Observe for availability of light.
Radiation[6]	Presence of radiation not to exceed 170 mrem in one year.	Have you ever lived for long periods of time at high altitudes (cosmic radiation)? Have you ever worked in places where radiation, carbon-14, or radon have been used? Have you worked in and about x-ray facilities? Have you ever had a radium implant or cobalt therapy? Have you spent long periods of your life around lead-based paints?

Physical System
5. Allergens and Toxins

CRITERIA	HEALTH STANDARDS	METHODS OF MEASUREMENT QUESTIONS, OBSERVATIONS, INSPECTIONS
Allergens[4]	Allergen counts not to exceed safe levels.	Are you allergic to air-borne allergens: Pollens? Dust? Mold? If so, what, if anything, have you done about it?

5. Allergens and Toxins (cont.)

CRITERIA	HEALTH STANDARDS	METHODS OF MEASUREMENT QUESTIONS, OBSERVATIONS, INSPECTIONS
	Ingredients or chemicals of food, serums and drugs are identified and labeled according to FDA regulations.	Do you obtain any of your food, medications or other drug supplies from sources other than FDA-regulated? If so, which ones?
Toxins	Any known toxins in natural environment are known and controlled.	Are there any likely poisonous substances in and about where you spend a lot of time, such as: Poisonous plants? Poisonous snakes? Bees? Insects? Are you particularly affected by any of these?

Physical System
6. Nutrients

CRITERIA	HEALTH STANDARDS	METHODS OF MEASUREMENT QUESTIONS, OBSERVATIONS, INSPECTIONS
Nutrients	Nutrients are available in sufficient quantity and quality to meet ADA	Every day, do you have available to you (and your family):

standards for each person.

Two or more cups of milk per day;

Two or more servings of meat, poultry, fish, eggs, dry peas, or nuts;

Four or more servings of whole grain, enriched or restored bread, or cereal;

Four or more servings among any of the following:

Citrus fruit;

A dark green or deep yellow vegetable;

Other vegetables, fruits, including potatoes.

If not, why not?

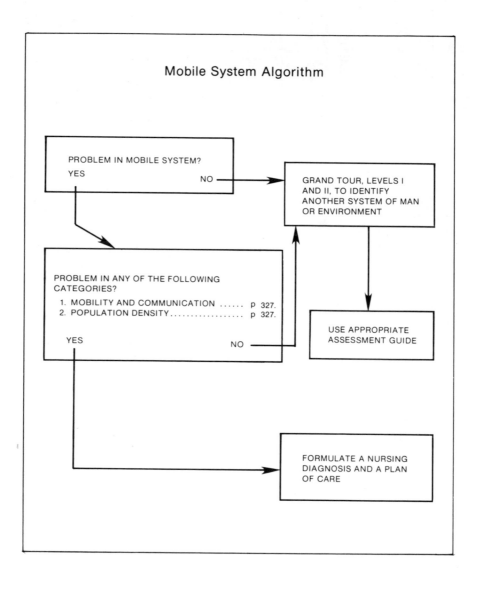

Mobile System Algorithm

PROBLEM IN MOBILE SYSTEM?
YES   NO

GRAND TOUR, LEVELS I AND II, TO IDENTIFY ANOTHER SYSTEM OF MAN OR ENVIRONMENT

PROBLEM IN ANY OF THE FOLLOWING CATEGORIES?
1. MOBILITY AND COMMUNICATION ...... p 327.
2. POPULATION DENSITY.................. p 327.

YES   NO

USE APPROPRIATE ASSESSMENT GUIDE

FORMULATE A NURSING DIAGNOSIS AND A PLAN OF CARE

Mobile System
1. Mobility and Communication

CRITERIA	HEALTH STANDARDS	METHODS OF MEASUREMENT QUESTIONS, OBSERVATIONS, INSPECTIONS
Mobility: Toffler,[7] — Increased automation results in increased forms of transportation. Sussman and Burchinal[8] — High-speed communication and transportation produce kin family networks.		
Culture: Mead[9] — Cultural values determine mode and frequency of mobility.		
Transportation	Availability of needed transport systems.	For the purposes of this book, specific methods of measurement derived from mobility and cultural theories have not been formulated.
Communication and transportation	Communication modes and transportation available to support kin family networks.	
Values	Consistency between cultural values and modes of mobility.	

Mobile System
2. Population Density

CRITERIA	HEALTH STANDARDS	METHODS OF MEASUREMENT QUESTIONS, OBSERVATIONS, INSPECTIONS
Spatial Relations: Rosow, S.[10] — Life space influences morale. One can predict what life-space environment will lead to good morale.		
Life space	Population density provides social contact as desired: limited, moderate, high.	For the purposes of this book, specific methods of measurement derived from spatial-relations theory have not been formulated.

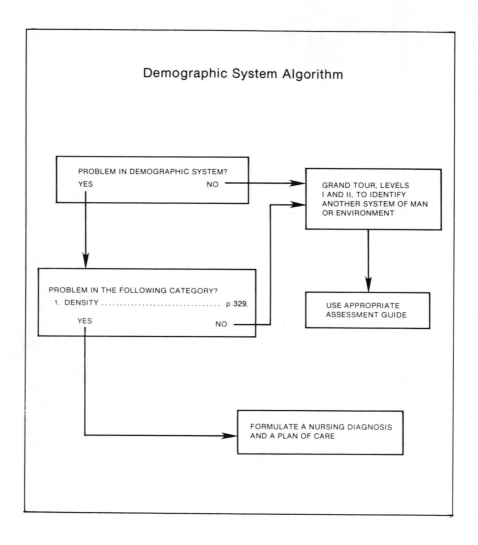

Demographic System Algorithm

PROBLEM IN DEMOGRAPHIC SYSTEM?

YES   NO

GRAND TOUR, LEVELS I AND II, TO IDENTIFY ANOTHER SYSTEM OF MAN OR ENVIRONMENT

PROBLEM IN THE FOLLOWING CATEGORY?

1. DENSITY .... p 329.

     YES   NO

USE APPROPRIATE ASSESSMENT GUIDE

FORMULATE A NURSING DIAGNOSIS AND A PLAN OF CARE

Demographic System
1. Density

CRITERIA	HEALTH STANDARDS	METHODS OF MEASUREMENT QUESTIONS, OBSERVATIONS, INSPECTIONS
Benarde[6] — Population density affects the quality of man's life.		
Density trends[11]		
Growth rate	A proportional birth/death rate not to exceed public health standards.	For the purposes of this book, specific methods of measurement derived from density theory have not been formulated.
Presymptomatic illness	Presence of presymptomatic illness and high-risk groups according to public health standards:	
	Blood pressure	
	Blood cholesterol	
	Blood sugar	
	Excessive poverty	
	Hereditary predisposition	
	Weight problems	
	Multiproblem families	
	Smoking	
	Drug abuse	
	Hazards	
Vulnerable/high-risk groups	Evidence of utilization of available health services for those identified as vulnerable or high-risk.	

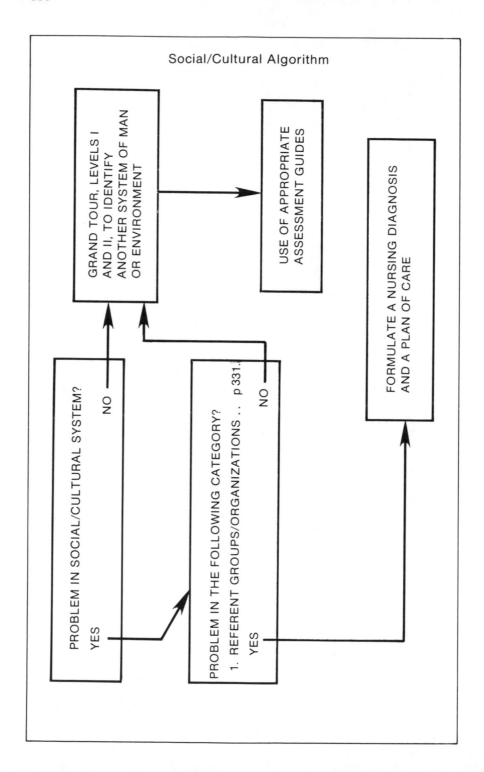

Social/Cultural Algorithm

Social-Cultural System
1. Referent Groups/Organizations

CRITERIA	HEALTH STANDARDS	METHODS OF MEASUREMENT QUESTIONS, OBSERVATIONS, INSPECTIONS
Ethnocentric Theory: Sumner[12] — The view of things in which one's own group is the center and all other groups are scaled and rated with reference to it.		
Referent group/s	Presence of at least one referent group with established norms and values.	For the purposes of this book, specific methods of measurement derived from ethnocentric and organizational theories have not been formulated.
Organization Theory: Lawrence and Lorsch[13] — Formal: For collective purposes to be achieved, formal organizations are necessary. Informal: For personal integrity, self-respect, and independence to be achieved, informal organizations are necessary.		
Organizations	Availability of formal and informal organizations designed to meet identified collective purposes and individualized social needs.	
Work processes.		
Social structure: hierarchies and interactions.		
Philosophy: values and beliefs.		
Authority relationships; rules, policies, and procedures.		

1. Referent Groups/Organizations *(cont.)*

CRITERIA	HEALTH STANDARDS	METHODS OF MEASUREMENT QUESTIONS, OBSERVATIONS, INSPECTIONS
Power balance		

Theories which interpret man as an interactive/affiliative system are also used to interpret the environment as a social/cultural system. The specific theories are: interpersonal, communication, group role, intimacy, and culture and appear on pages 302-308.

References

1. Spencer M: *Contemporary Economics.* 2nd ed, New York, Worth Publishers Inc, 1974, pp 4, 20, 21.
2. McCool B, Brown M: *The Management Response: Conceptual, Technical, and Human Skills of Health Administration.* Philadelphia, WB Saunders Co, 1977, p 11.
3. Archer S, Fleshman M: *Community Health Nursing, Patterns and Practice.* North Scituate, Mass, Duxbury Press, 1975, p 176.
4. Beland I, Passos J: *Clinical Nursing: Pathophysiological and Psychosocial Approaches.* 3rd ed, New York, Macmillan Publishing Co, Inc, 1975, pp 55, 306-319.
5. Sutterly D, Donnally G: *Perspectives in Human Development, Nursing Through The Life Cycle.* Philadelphia, JB Lippincott Co, 1973, pp 272-275.
6. Benarde M: *Our Precarious Habitat.* New York, WC Norton and co, Inc, 1973, pp 232-236, 378.
7. Toffler A: *Future Shock.* New York, Random House, 1970, pp 74-94.
8. Sussman MB, Burchinal L: Kin family network: Unheralded structure in current conceptualizations of family functioning. *Marriage and Family Living* 24:3, August 1962.
9. Mead M (ed): *Cultural Patterns and Technical Change.* UNESCO, New York, A Mentor Book, 1955, pp 12-13.
10. Rosow S: Housing and local ties of the aged. *Patterns of Living and Housing of Middle-Aged and Older People: Proceedings of Research Conference.* Washington, DC, Department of Health, Education, and Welfare, 1965, pp 45-57.
11. Freeman R: *Community Health Nursing Practice.* Philadelphia, WB Saunders Co, 1970, pp 254-256.
12. Sumner W: *Folkways.* New York, Ginn, 1906, pp 12-13.
13. Lawrence P, Lorsch J: *Developing Organizations: Diagnosis and Action.* Menlo Park, Calif. Addison-Wesley Publishing Co, Inc, 1969, pp 1-22, 62-71.

APPENDIX C
Selected Assessment Guides

SELECTED ASSESSMENT GUIDES

Appendix C contains several selected assessment guides or nursing histories, similar to many in actual use. None of them purports to articulate a theory base clearly; but any of them can easily be revised to do so.

1. **Nursing History, Acute Care.** This represents a very general systems review. Two of its categories, "Emotional Status" and "Apparent or Revealed Deficits," use key words that relate man's psychological and sensory/perceptive systems. It concludes by guiding the nurse to tentative conclusions.

2. **Health History Guide, General.** This form guides the nurse through a complete body-systems review. It reminds the nurse to obtain information about the patient's emotional or psychological status, and his family situation.

3. **The Physical Examination Guide.** This provides a detailed checklist for assessing all the body systems. It is designed to be used in conjunction with a more general health-history guide for a comprehensive assessment.

4. **Nursing History, Hospitalization.** This is a typical, brief data-gathering guide that attends to safety, comfort, and security needs.

5. **Neurological Assessment Criteria and Guidelines for Clinical Nursing Practice.** This form is an example of a specialized assessment guide generally used in an intensive care setting. It includes a checklist of physiological parameters that should be assessed at periodic intervals.

6. **Psychological Assessment.** This is a general outline which can be used to guide one through a psychological assessment. It is designed to aid the nurse in evaluating several aspects of man: cognitive/intellectual, sensory/perceptive, and psychological.

7. **The Nursing Discharge Plan.** This plan is included here because it represents an assessment guide for the end phase of patient care. This particular guide is designed to double as a referral form.

8. **Human Needs Assessment Scale.** This scale presents a different approach to assessment. It lists those factors that should be assessed. For each factor, statements describing poor, minimal, and good responses allow the nurse to make evaluative judgments regarding the patient's status.

9. **Nursing History, Extended Care.** This form is a good example of an assessment guide that focuses on the client's preferences and daily routines. Elements of this guide reflect some relationship to psychological, sensory/perceptive, physiological, and mobility theories.
10. **Guidelines for Community Assessment.** This guide focuses on the community, or on the environment, as client. Implicit in many of its elements are certain environmental systems: demographic, mobile, and social/cultural.

1. Nursing History, Acute Care

NAME _____ DATE OF HISTORY _____

DIAGNOSIS _____ DATE OF ADMISSION _____

AGE _____ SEX _____ BIRTHDATE _____

OCCUPATION _____ RECREATIONAL INTEREST ____

PRIOR HOSPITALIZATIONS:

WHEN _____ WHERE _____ DIAGNOSIS _____

ABILITY TO UNDERSTAND QUESTIONS AND IDEAS:

EMOTIONAL STATUS (CHECK APPROPRIATE AND EXPLAIN)
Anxious
Depressed
Aggressive
Regressed
Other
Effect of Illness on self-image
Ability to relate   Attention span:

APPARENT OR REVEALED DEFICITS
Hearing
Sight
Touch
Smell
Taste
Movement
Equilibrium

SKIN CONDITION
Dehydrated
Edema
Discoloration   Where:
Broken areas   Where:
Cleanliness   Where:

Localized temperature changes
Preference for bathing
Hair, nail care
Special back care

REASON FOR ADMISSION: EXPECTED LENGTH OF STAY

NUTRITION

Condition of mouth & teeth
Dentures
Oral hygiene
Appetite   How many meals _____
Food — Likes
        Dislikes   Snacks _____
Fluid — Likes
        Dislikes   Meal patterns
Allergies   What frequency _____
Use of alcoholic beverages

ELIMINATION

Bowel habits
Laxatives   Kind used _____
Urination   Frequency _____
  Frequency   Catheter _____
  Amount
  Color
  Pain
  Retention

REST AND SLEEP PATTERN

Naps
Bedtime   When _____   How long _____
Easily disturbed?   Waking time _____
Device for getting to sleep? Up at night _____

HISTORY OF PAIN

Location
Devices used to relieve
Analgesics used

ADL ASSISTANCE REQUIRED

None ☐   Minimal ☐   Moderate ☐   Full ☐
Bathing   Toileting
Dressing   Transferring
Feeding   Walking

TENTATIVE CONCLUSIONS

UNDERSTANDING OF ILLNESS:

UNDERSTANDING OF PHYSICIAN'S TREATMENT PLAN:

MEANINGFUL OTHERS:

USUAL DAILY ACTIVITIES:

OBSERVATIONS MADE WHILE TAKING HISTORY:

ITEMS NEEDING FURTHER INVESTIGATION:

2. Health History Guide, General*

1. SOURCE AND IDENTIFICATION INFORMATION
   NAME: _____ DATE: _____ AGE: ____ SEX: ____
   MEDICAL RECORD OR SOCIAL SECURITY NO. _____
   DATE OF BIRTH: _____ PLACE OF BIRTH: _____
   ADDRESS: _____
   EMPLOYER AND BUSINESS ADDRESS: _____
   SPOUSE EMPLOYER: _____

2. CHIEF COMPLAINT (IN SUBJECT'S OWN WORDS, WHY HE HAS COME TODAY)

3. HISTORY OF PRESENTING ILLNESS (NARRATIVE FORMAT)

   CHRONOLOGICAL DEVELOPMENT OF PATIENT'S PROBLEM (USE DATES). DATE OF ONSET.
   a. What brings it on?
   b. How does it start? Relationship to any activity.
   c. Nature of symptom: i.e., pain: sharp, dull, intermittent, radiating, aching, where, effect on daily living.
   d. What has subject done at home regarding symptom and effect?
   e. Previous treatment? Effectiveness?
   f. Family members with same problem?
   g. Pertinent negatives

---

*Courtesy of James Comins, R.N., M.S., Katherine Jones, R.N., M.S., California State University, Sacramento, Division of Nursing.

    h. Related symptoms
    i. Patient perception of cause?
    j. Expectations of care?

4. PATIENT PROFILE (PATIENT AS PERSON)
    a. Occupation (note environmental hazards)
    b. Job satisfaction — job potential — income level
    c. Level of education
    d. Home ownership — rental — shared quarters
    e. Marital status — number and ages of children
    f. Number and ages of other dependents
    g. Community life/activities
    h. Recreational and/or social activities
    i. Sexual function
    j. Dietary preferences
    k. Travel
    l. Present habits
        1. Drinking patterns
        2. Smoking or tobacco usage
        3. Exercise pattern
        4. Sleep pattern
        5. Elimination pattern
        6. Drugs taken at home
        7. Dental health

EMOTIONAL OR PSYCHOLOGICAL STATUS

Encourage patient to verbalize feelings about life satisfactions, inter-personal relations with family, superiors, co-workers, peers, and so forth. Note present adjustment to life/societal situation.

Include typical 24-hour day and 24-hour diet history.

5. PAST MEDICAL HISTORY

(Chronic diseases frequently are a development of previous acute illnesses. History also tells how the patient has reacted to past illnesses.)

(Use the following outline as a guide in exploring past medical history.)
    a. General level of health as seen by the patient.
    b. Childhood diseases: mumps; measles; chicken pox; whooping cough; scarlet fever; diphtheria; poliomyelitis; rheumatic fever; tonsillitis. Seek date, symptoms, results of treatment, and complications.
    c. Immunications: DPT; polio; measles; typhoid; influenza; others. Any reactions?
    d. Allergies: medications; ASA, PCN; Sulfa; Iodine; foods; animals; dust; pollen; others. Give nature of any reaction along with time course. What type of treatment given? Any complications?

e. Medical diseases: dates; where treated; complications.
f. Surgeries: date; procedure; where done; any complications.
g. Trauma: date; where treated; what happened; complications.
h. Psychiatric treatment; date; where; what; complications.
i. Obstetrical history:

> Age at menarche, frequency, duration of periods, estimated flow (how many pads and how much saturated in one day)
>> Number of pregnancies
>> Number of live births
>> Number of miscarriages and therapeutic abortions

6. FAMILY HISTORY

Age and present health status of parents, grandparents, and siblings. If deceased, give date, age, and cause of death. Include family history of congenital or acquired disease: i.e., diabetes, heart disease, stroke, kidney disease, cancer, hypertension, mental illness.

(May draw family tree. Include key to explain symbols.)

7. REVIEW OF SYSTEMS (ELABORATE ON POSITIVE SYMP-TOMS OR REFER TO APPROPRIATE SECTION OF HISTORY: 0 = NEGATIVE: V = POSITIVE.) (MAY USE THIS FORM)

Head:	__headaches	__facial pain	
	__head injury		
Eyes:	__diplopia	__vision loss	__pain
	__redness	__glaucoma	__infection
Ears:	__hearing loss		__earache
	__discharge	__tinnitus	__vertigo
Nose:	__obstruction	__bleeding	__discharge (nature of)
	__sneezing	__hay fever	__sinusitis
Mouth:	__sore mouth	__sore tongue	__dental caries
	__bleeding gums	__sore throat	__loss of taste
Neck:	__hoarseness	__dysphagia	__goiter
	__pain	__stiffness	__lumps or nodes
Lungs:	__wheeze	__cough	__sputum
	__hemoptysis	__bronchitis	__pneumonia
	__pleurisy	__asthma	__TB

Lungs: Date of last chest x-ray _____
__SOB   __dyspnea (Describe occupational history if related to pulmonary status.)

Heart:	__SOB	__orthopnea	__paroxysmal nocturnal dyspnea

___palpitations   ___edema   ___rheumatic
                                      fever
___heart murmurs ___hypertension   ___heart attack
___cyanosis (central or peripheral)

Breasts: ___breast lumps
           ___discharge from nipple
           ___increased vascularity of breasts
           ___asymmetrical breasts

G.I.:   ___anorexia   ___nausea
           ___vomiting   ___constipation
           ___diarrhea   ___pain
           ___bleeding   ___jaundice
           ___"tarry stools" ___ulcer
           ___gallbladder disease

G.V.:   ___frequency   ___polyuria
           ___nocturia   ___dysuria
           ___hematuria   ___difficulty starting or stopping the
                              urinary stream
           ___incontinence   ___urinary tract
           ___infections   ___stones
           ___hernia   ___spyhilis
           ___gonorrhea, or other venereal disease

GYN: ___menses
           ___frequency
           ___amount of flow
           ___pain   intermenstrual bleeding
           ___vaginal discharge
           ___purititis
           ___symptoms related to menopause if appropriate

OB: Number of pregnancies _____
           Number of live births _____
           Number of living children _____
           ___Obstetrical complications

PERIPHERAL VASCULAR:
           ___varicose veins ___phlebitis   ___cramps with
           ___stasis ulcers   exercise (intermit-
           ___history of   tent claudication)
           frostbite
           ___skin reaction to
           cold

Neurological:
           ___seizures (describe aura, length of time it lasts, behavior
           during seizure, date of onset, frequency, and medications)
           ___faints

    ___ptosis
    ___gait
    ___weakness or paralysis
    ___paresthesias
    ___tremor
    ___numbness

Skin: ___rashes   ___nodule   ___sores
         ___bruises   ___change in texture or color
         ___moles   (i.e., vitiligo)
         ___scars

Blood: ___anemia   ___bleeding tendencies
         ___transfusion history

Endocrine:
    ___diabetes or its symptoms (weakness, dehydration, poly-
    dipsia, polyuria, polyphagia)
    ___thyroid trouble
    ___recent weight changes

The intent of the review of systems is to check the subject's health status in head-to-toe fashion. This serves to sum up the medical history and jog the subject's memory. Since he/she may think of something significant at the end of the ROS, it is appropriate to ask the subject if he/she has thought of anything else which he/she wants to tell the interviewer.

The physical examination will logically follow as further exploration of the patient's physical status.

PHYSICAL EXAMINATION†

LABORATORY DATA

Each agency will determine own laboratory base data. Recommendations for minimum laboratory data are: CBC, serology, urinalysis, chest x-ray, and electrocardiogram. For clients/patients forty plus can be added: vital capacity and peak flow measurements, tonometry, blood glucose, cholesterol, uric acid, calcium, blood urea nitrogen or creatinine, total protein with albumin/globulin ratio, electrolytes, pap smear.

---

†*The physical examination guide appears next in this appendix.*

3. PHYSICAL EXAMINATION GUIDE**

1. GENERAL INSPECTION
   A. Begin the examination of the patient by observing him from the first moment you see him, and make introductions. Continue observations systematically yet subtly, while interviewing the patient and taking his health history. After the interview, it is useful to initiate physical contact by taking the patient's vital signs and examining his hands — maneuvers which are relatively non-threatening.
   B. During the "General Inspection," note the following:

	Examples of Abnormalities
1. Apparent state of health.	1. Frail, acutely or chronically ill.
2. Signs of distress; i.e., cardio-respiratory, pain, anxiety.	2. SOB, cough, anxious or pained facial expression, cold, moist palms, fidgety movements.
3. Skin color	3. Pallor, cyanosis, jaundice.
4. Stature and habitus: measure height, note body build, body proportions, gross deformities.	4. Long limbs in proportion to trunk in hypogonadism.
5. Weight: weigh, note if obese or thin for particular body build.	5. Obesity
6. Posture, motor activity, gait.	6. Slumped posture, tremors, ataxia.
7. Dress, grooming, personal hygiene.	7. Unkempt appearance in depression.
8. Odors: of breath or body	8. Breath odor with alcohol, diabetes (acetone), pulmonary infections.
9. Facial expression: at rest and in interaction with others.	9. Anxiety, depression, pain, apathy.
10. Manner, mood, relationships to other persons and things.	10. Uncooperativeness, hostility, distrustfulness.

**Courtesy of Marilyn Hopkins, R.N., M.S., California State University, Sacramento, Division of Nursing.*

11. Speech: pace, pitch, clarity.

11. Fast speech with hyperthyroidism, dysphasia.

12. State of awareness, consciousness: include speed of response to questions and apparent comprehension.

12. Inattentiveness, drowsiness, stupor, coma.

13. Vital signs: T, P, R, BP.

13. Fever, tachycardia, tachypnea, hypotension.

2. SKIN

A. Inspect and palpate, noting:
1. Color
2. Vascularity, evidence of bleeding and bruising
3. Lesions: identify color, type, grouping, and distribution
4. Edema
5. Moisture
6. Temperature: feel with back of fingers
7. Texture
8. Mobility (ease of skin movement)
9. Turgor (speed of skin returning to place)
10. Inspect and palpate fingernails and toenails: note color, shape and lesions.

3. HEAD AND NECK

A. Hair: Quantity, distribution, texture
B. Scalp: Scaliness, lumps, lesions
C. Skull: Size and contour, deformities, lumps, tenderness
D. Face: Facial expression, symmetry, involuntary movements, edema, masses
E. Skin: Color pigmentation, texture, thickness, hair distribution, lesions
F. Eyes:
1. Visual Acuity: Read printed words, count fingers, distinguish light from dark, one eye at a time.
2. Position and alignment
3. Eyebrows: Quantity, distribution, scaliness
4. Eyelids: Edema, redness, lesions, condition and direction of eyelashes
5. Conjunctiva and Sclera: Note color, nodules, swelling
6. Pupils: Size, shape, equality, reaction to light, pupillary accommodation
7. Convergence of eyes with near vision
8. With the ophthalmoscope, visualize the retina (orange-red round or oval structure), optic disc (orange-white), veins

(dark red), and arterioles (light red). Use right hand and right eye to examine patient's right eye with the ophthalmoscope. Reverse is true for examination of the patient's left eye.

G. Ears
  1. Deformities, lumps, lesions
  2. Pain, discharge, inflammation
  3. Examine with otoscope
     a. Tip head slightly to opposite side
     b. Pull auricle up, back and slightly outward
     c. Insert largest speculum that canal will tolerate. Position slightly downward and forward.
     d. Identify wax, discharge, foreign bodies in ear canal. Note redness, swelling.
     e. Identify eardrum (silvery and shiny).
  4. Hearing Acuity
     a. Occlude one ear at a time and standing 1-2 feet from patient softly whisper numbers. Obstruct patient's vision of your mouth while you speak to prevent lip-reading.
  5. Weber Test
     a. Put base of lightly vibrating tuning fork on top of head or middle of forehead. Sound normally perceived in midline or equally in both ears.
  6. Rinne Test: Compare conduction of sound through air and bone.
     a. Place lightly vibrating tuning fork on mastoid process until patient can no longer hear sound. Then quickly place vibrating fork near ear canal, its side toward the ear. Note how long patient can hear the sound. Sound normally heard longer through air than bone.

H. Nose and Sinuses
  1. Inspect nose for deformity, asymmetry
  2. Insert short, side nasal speculum and check for color, swelling, exudate, bleeding (nasal muscosa redder than oral mucosa).
  3. Nasal Septum: Bleeding, perforation, deviation
  4. Palpate for sinus tenderness: Front sinus (below eyebrow) maxillary sinus (medially below cheek bone).

I. Mouth and Pharynx
  1. Remove dentures, if present, before this part of the examination.
  2. Lips: Color, moisture, lumps, ulcers, cracking.
  3. Buccal Mucosa: With flashlight and tongue blade, inspect for

color, pigmentation, ulcers, nodules (patchy pigmentation is normal in Negroes).

4. Gums and Teeth: Discoloration, swelling, bleeding gums, loose or carious teeth.
5. Roof of Mouth: Color, architecture of hard palate.
6. Tongue: Symmetry (12th cranial nerve), white patches, nodules, ulcerations, varicose veins.
   a. Nodules, ulcerations found anywhere in the mouth should be palpated with a gloved finger. Thickening (infiltration of tissues) may indicate malignancy.
7. Pharynx: Note rise of soft palate when patient says "ah-h-h" (10th cranial nerve), check uvula and tonsils for edema, redness, exudate.

J. Neck
   1. Note symmetry, masses, trachea midline.
   2. Palpate lymph nodes: In front and behind ears, under mandible, down sides of neck under ear.
      a. Tender nodes suggest inflammation, while hard or fixed nodes suggest malignancy.
   3. Palpate thyroid

K. Thorax and Lungs
   1. Inspect chest shape (A-P diameter) slope of ribs, abnormal retraction of interspaces during inspiration, rate and rhythm of breathing.
   2. Palpate areas which are tender or abnormal in appearance.
   3. Fremitus: Palpable vibrations from the bronchopulmonary system to the chest wall when patient says "gg" or "l".
      a. Decreased with soft voice, obstructed bronchus, pleural space occupied by fluid, air, or solid tissue.
      b. Increased over large bronchi and over consolidated (more dense) lung tissue.
   4. Percuss side to side both lungs.
      a. Normal lung — "resonant" sounds (loud in intensity and low pitched).
      b. Fluid in lungs — "dull" sounds (medium in intensity and pitch).
   5. Auscultate breath sounds (B.S.)
      a. Normal B.S.
         1. Vesicular (insp, exp) — most of lungs
         2. Bronchovesicular (insp, exp) — near mainstream bronchi
         3. Bronchial (insp, exp) — over trachea

   b. Abnormal B.S.

    1. Rales: Sound of air through fluid

     a. Fine rales: In smaller air passages

     b. Coarse rales: In larger air passages; i.e., trachea, bronchi (Classified by some sources as rhonchi).

    2. Rhonchi: Sound of air flowing through narrowed passages.

     a. Musical or sibilant (wheezes): Originate in small air passages, high-pitched.

     b. Sonorous Rhonchi: Usually with obstruction of bronchi or trachea, low-pitched, snoring sound.

    3. Pleural friction rubs: Crackling, grating sounds originating in an inflamed pleura.

L. Heart

  1. Inspect: Venous distention in neck, pulsations over aorta, pulmonary artery, right and left ventricles.

  2. Palpate: Neck veins, peripheral pulses (carotid, brachial, radial, femoral, popliteal, pedal), PMI.

  3. Auscultate: Normal heart sounds, murmurs, gallops, pericardial rubs.

M. Breasts and Axillae

  1. Inspect and palpate for masses

N. Abdomen: Note exception to rule of order for doing a P.E. (Inspect, auscultate, palpate, percuss).

  1. Inspect: Scars, stretch marks, dilated veins, rashes, lesions, umbilicus, contour.

  2. Auscultate: Bowel sounds.

  3. Palpate: Masses, tenderness, rigidity, enlarged organs, hernias, ascites.

  4. Percuss: To determine size of abdominal organs, air in stomach and bowel.

   a. Stomach — resonant

   b. Liver — dull

O. Male genitalia and hernias

P. Female genitalia

Q. Neurologic

  1. Mental status and speech

  2. Cranial nerves

   a. I (Olfactory): Smell

   b. II (Optic): Visual acuity

   c. III, IV, VI (Oculomotor, Trochlear, Abducens): Pupil

reactions, eye movements.

    1. Have patient follow your finger with his eyes, either horizontal, vertical, or rotary.
    2. Nystagmus: Involuntary oscillation of the eye, either horizontal, vertical, or rotary.
    3. Check pupillary reflexes.
    4. Check for lid-lag.

d. V, VII (Trigeminal, Facial): Facial sensation and motor function.

    1. Stroke face with fingers or use pin pricks.
    2. Have patient wrinkle forehead, smile, close eyes tightly so you can't open them, puff out his cheeks, clench his teeth.

e. VIII (Acoustic): Hearing

    1. Whisper, ticking watch, fingers rubbing by individual ears.

f. IX, X (Glossopharyngeal and Vagus): Lifting of soft palate, gag reflex, coordinated swallowing, speech without hoarseness.

g. XI (Spinal Accessory): Shoulder and neck muscles.

    1. Have patient shrug shoulders, bend neck.

h. XII (Hypoglossal): Tongue

    1. Have patient stick out tongue.

3. Motor System

    a. Normal gait
    b. Walk heel to toe
    c. Stand with feet together, arms down, with eyes open and then closed (Romberg Test)
    d. Note strength, atrophy, tremors, or fasciculations

4. Sensory System

    a. Pain
    b. Temperature
    c. Light touch
    d. Vibration
    e. Position (proprioception)
    f. Discriminative sensation

5. Reflexes

    a. Biceps
    b. Triceps
    c. Brachioradialis
    d. Abdominal
    e. Cremasteric (Scrotal)
    f. Knee

g. Ankle
h. Babinski
i. Reflexes graded on a 0 to 4+ scale:
1. 4+ very brisk, hyperactive
2. 3+ brisker than average
3. 2+ average, normal
4. 1+ diminished, low normal
5. 0 - no response

4. Nursing History, Hospitalization

NAME: _____ AGE: _____ SEX: ____

ADMITTED: _____

REASON: _____

HOW: _____

GENERAL PHYSICAL DESCRIPTION:

PRIOR HOSPITAL EXPERIENCES:

When:

Why:

What did you feel about it? (Likes and dislikes)

CURRENT HOSPITAL EXPERIENCE:

What led to your coming to the hospital?

What could be done to make you most comfortable?

Are you expecting visitors?

Are there any limitations you would like placed on visitors?

PERSONAL HISTORY AND HABITS:

Occupation:	Hobbies/Recreation:	Prostheses:
Education:	Smoking:	
Family Unit:	Allergies:	

Has illness changed your normal daily routine? If so, how?

| Elimination habits: | Bathing habits: |
| Sleeping habits: | Eating and fluid intake habits: |

SAFETY NEEDS: (SPECIFIC)

Present needs:

Potential needs:

MEDICATIONS TAKEN ROUTINELY:

NURSING OBSERVATIONS: (INDICATE PATTERN OF COM-
MUNICATIONS AND EMOTIONAL REACTIONS)

5. Neurological Assessment Criteria and Guidelines for Clinical Nursing Practice‡

These guidelines and criteria for coding on the assessment guide will be helpful in developing an action-planning type of nursing assessment.

1. GENERAL CRITERIA
   A. This assessment tool is designed to assist the nurse in gathering data on which the documentation in the nurse's notes is based. It is not an hourly flow sheet or graph record for vital signs, but rather reflects a baseline functioning for the patient. At the beginning of each shift an assessment should be made. Subsequent entries during a shift would be made only when changes occur.
   B. Indicate that a problem exists in an assessed area with a (+) and indicate that there is no problem with a (-). Actual numerical values (i.e., BP, T, P, etc.) may be recorded initially to support existence of a problem.

2. RESPIRATORY-CIRCULATION STATUS
   A. Check rate, depth, character (deep and stertorous or Cheyne-Stokes), check expansion, and position for most effective respiration (semi-prone position or thirty degrees aids in drainage of secretions and in keeping tongue forward); never let head slump on the chest.
   B. Note origin, amount, and character of secretions (changes in rate, character, etc. of respirations may be indicative of mucous plugs or increasing intracranial pressure); pharyngeal secretions can be aspirated safely to prevent swallowed accumulation which leads to vomiting.
   C. Watch pulse pressure differences; check quality of pulse (full and bounding, slight irregularity), muscle spasms can give false highs in blood pressure readings; increased intracranial pressure occurs when there is a sharp increase in blood pressure and a decrease in pulse rate; circulatory collapse occurs when there is a sharp decrease in blood pressure with an increase in pulse rate and respirations.
   D. Check skin (temperature, color, general appearance, pressure areas).

‡*Courtesy of Robyn Nelson, R.N., M.S., California State University, Sacramento, Division of Nursing.*

4. NEUROMUSCULAR STATUS
   A. Level of consciousness
      1. Degree of responsiveness:
         1+ = No response to stimuli
         2+ = Comatose with response to stimuli
         3+ = Reacts to pain stimuli with purposeful withdrawal movements and verbal responses, but with no conversation
         4+ = Is responsive, arousing when stimulated and replying appropriately to commands
         5+ = Patient is awake and answering questions appropriately, and is oriented to person, place, time, and events (memory).
   B. Perceptual responses assessment (sight, hearing, taste, smell, touch, or tactile pressure, temperature, pain).
   C. Assess patient understanding of verbal commands (ability to obey, answer to name, have verbal expression, and cooperate).
   D. Pupillary status assessment (size, dilatation, equality, reactivity); differentiate between sleep and coma, for in normal sleep pupils are always constricted.
   E. Gag, corneal, or Babinski reflexes (normal or abnormal).
   F. Speech responses (clear, none, slurred, slow or quick, appropriate statements, meaningful, attentive).
   G. Motion and strength of extremities (equality of sides in mobility and strength, lethargy, muscle tone).
   H. Involuntary movements (jerking of the head, tremors of the eyelids or mouth, seizure activity, rigidity, flaccidity, joint mobility, vomiting, incontinence, presence or absence of decerebrate posturing).
   I. Voluntary movements (gait, performance of skilled or purposeful sets, proprioception ataxia).

5. MEDICATIONS (describe the effects of on the various body systems)

A NEUROLOGICAL GUIDE FOR NURSING ASSESSMENT

NAME: _____ PHYSICIAN: _____

DIAGNOSIS: _____ ROOM #: _____

(+) Indicates problem (-) No problem

DATE TIME								
Parameters								
BP								
T								
P								

R									
Breathing Rhythm									
Venous Pressure									
Skin Color									
Intake									
Output									
Pupil Reactions									
Pupils									
Eyes and Related Movements									
Ptosis of eyelids									
Periocular edema									
Disconjugation									
Headache									
Level of Consciousness									
Orientation									
Person									
Place									
Object									
Event									
Arousability — Responses, Stimuli									
Pain									
Tactile									
Verbal									
Motor Responses									
Involuntary movements									
Voluntary movements									
Neck stiffness									
Rigidity									
Speech									
Abnormal reflexes									
Bilateral hand grips									
Restlessness									
Agitation									

Lethargy								
Gait								
Medications								
Effects on systems								

6. Psychological Assessment

1. APPEARANCE, ATTITUDE, AND ACTIVITY
   A. General physical appearance
   B. State of health
   C. Manner mobility
   D. Facial expression
   E. Appropriateness of dress
   F. Character of motor activities, perseveration
   G. Reaction to examiner

2. SENSORIUM AND INTELLIGENCE
   A. Orientation
   B. Memory
   C. Abstractive ability
   D. Intelligence level
   E. Insight
   F. Judgment

3. THOUGHT PROCESSES
   A. Productivity, spontaneity
   B. Coherence and continuity of thought, associations
   C. Blocking, mutism, echolalia

4. THOUGHT CONTENT
   A. Preoccupations, hallucinations, illusions, delusions

5. EMOTIONAL STATE
   A. Affect, mood, appropriateness, and lability

1. APPEARANCE, ATTITUDE AND ACTIVITY

The items from *a* to *g* all are observable characteristics of the patient. Be careful of subjective interpretations here. For example, item *e*, Appropriateness of dress; if you find yourself disapproving of a particular dress, you may say that an individual is inappropriately dressed and yet this may be appropriate dress for his life-style. So, the appearance, attitudes, and activities should relate to the history and background of the patient.

2. SENSORIUM AND INTELLIGENCE
   a. Orientation (time, place, person). Orientation refers to patient sense of time, place and who he is.
   b. Memory. There are three levels of memory; remote, recent, and immediate, or short-term memory. Remote memory has to do with all those past events that occurred more than a week ago. Recent memory has to do with memory within the last several hours to a day. This would include questions like, "What did you have for lunch yesterday?" and a test of having the patient listen to the names of three objects and then having him repeat them after ten minutes of the interview. Immediate or short-term memory has to do with the recall of numbers given to a patient, having him repeat numbers 1-2-3-4, either forward or in reverse. Also, doing serial sevens, subtracting 7 from 100 and continuing to subtract 7 in a series involves the testing of short-term memory.

   Short-term memory is generally interfered when there is drug abuse, such as use of marijuana, or when a person is preoccupied with depressive thoughts over delusions. Intermediate-range memory is usually interfered when there is some form of organic problem such as alcoholic hallucinosis, or Korsakoff's Psychosis. Note that in Korsakoff's Psychosis, confabulation may be used to fill in the missing memory. Loss of remote memory is seen only in severely impaired individuals, either toxic or functional.
   c. Abstractive ability. The testing of abstraction is important in diagnosing psychotic thinking. Psychotics are generally unable to abstract. Abstraction means the ability to flow from a concrete type of thinking to a philosophical type of thinking. Psychotics think only concretely and lack the ability to abstract. Proverb interpretation and similarities both test abstract ability.
   d. Intelligence level. Vocabulary, sentence structure, and period of time spent in education are all indices of intelligence level.
   e. Insight. Insight refers to the person's psychological awareness of himself. Does he see himself as having a problem? Does he realize that there are other psychological awareness forces at work on him?
   f. Judgment. Judgment is a function of the frontal lobes. It is the newest part of man's brain, and is very sensitive to drugs and toxins. Judgment may be evaluated by observing the individual's reaction to his current situation, or asking specific questions such as: "Why is it better to build a house of brick than of wood?"

3. THOUGHT PROCESSES
   Thought processes literally mean the way thoughts proceed through an individual's brain. That may be tested in the following manner:
   a. *Productivity* and *spontaneity* are judged by the ease and rate with which an individual answers any questions posed to him. It is

also evaluated during the earlier part of the examination when a patient is giving a history.

b. *Coherence* and *continuity* of thought can only be evaluated through speech. Therefore, you are looking at coherence and continuity of speech, how sentences hang together, whether or not conclusions are reached in sentences, and whether or not they relate to the subject at hand. All reflect continuity of thought.

c. *Blocking* is a difficulty in recalling. It may also be an interruption of the train of thought or speech that you can see is due to emotional factors, such as anxiety. Echolalia is the repetition of the patient's own words or words that you say as an examiner. Both these phenomena are easily observable during the earlier part of an intake interview.

4. THOUGHT CONTENT

Thought content is tested on the assumption that someone needs psychiatric treatment because they have got into a mental rut.

In increasing order of severity you will observe the following phenomenon of mental focusing: *Preoccupations* means focus on one or two general areas of thoughts. These may appear as repetitive dreams, daytime fantasies, or thoughts that "I just can't get off my mind." *Delusion* is the focus on a false belief that is basically out of keeping with the individual's level of knowledge and is maintained against logical argument. Delusions may be of grandeur (exaggerated ideas of one's importance), of persecution (ideas that one has been singled out for persecution), or of reference (incorrect assumptions that certain casual or unrelated remarks, or the behaviors of others, apply to one's self). An *illusion* is the focus on a misinterpretation of a real external sensory experience. *Hallucination* is the focus on a false sensory perception in the absence of an actual external stimulus. An hallucination may occur in any one of the five senses.

5. EMOTIONAL STATE

Emotional state is the way in which emotions or feelings "flow." The *affect* is a psychiatric term for the mood or emotional tone. It is called *flattened* when there is an abnormally small range of emotional expression. It is called *labile* when there is a rapidly shifting emotional state. It is called *inappropriate* when emotional expressions are not in accord with the situation, or with what is being said.

The following are additional terms used in psychiatric jargon that should be clearly understood:

Autism: A state of thinking in which the sensitive personal boundary or barrier is lost. Therefore, the person believes that other people or things can impinge on his personal private space and that he also may have ability to extend himself beyond his own personal private space.

An example is the individual that thinks electronic beams are trying to control him.

Confabulation: A defensive "filling in" of actual memory gaps by imaginary of fantasied experiences. They are often complex and are recounted in a detailed and plausible way as though they were factual.

Circumstantial: A characteristic of conversation that proceeds indirectly to its goal idea with many tedious details and parenthetical and irrelevent additions.

Neologism: A new word or condensed combination of several words coined by a patient to express a highly complex meaning related to his own experiences or complex.

Phobia: An obsessive persistent unrealistic fear of an external object or situation.

7. Nursing Discharge Plan

This plan is a brief summary of the patient's progress while hospitalized. Its purpose is to orient the visiting nurse to the patient's situation so she can provide uninterrupted care.

PROCEDURE:

1. All three shifts are to add to the discharge plan. This plan will be discussed and written during report times.
2. Social worker will notify visiting nurse of patient's discharge.
3. Visiting nurse will contact unit to discuss the discharge plan with staff nurse.
4. Written nursing discharge plan accompanies doctor's discharge plan.

PATIENT'S NAME:_____ MED. REC. NO. _____

ADDRESS _____

DIAGNOSIS_____ DATE _____

1. EMOTIONAL NEEDS
   A. Patient's understanding of illness

   B. Stage of illness (check one and explain briefly)
      1. Denial/Shock
      2. Anger
      3. Negotiation
      4. Adjustment
      5. Acceptance

2. PHYSICAL NEEDS
   A. Extent of self-management

   B. Possible problem areas

   C. Materials or resource services needed

3. SOCIAL NEEDS
   A. Family situation (physical and social environment)
   B. Family members in the household, or other available assistance
   C. Family's emotional response to illness
4. SPECIAL COMFORT OR DAILY ROUTINE NEEDS

5. GENERAL DESCRIPTION OF PATIENT, INTERACTIONAL PATTERNS, AND LIFE STYLE

358

8. Human Needs Assessment Scale*

PHYSICAL	POOR 1	MINIMAL 2	GOOD 3
1. Good skin color, no cyanosis.	Ashen or cyanotic + ashen.	Pale or ashen but no cyanosis.	Warm skin; no cyanosis.
2. Freedom from sense of fatigue; energy to carry out life activities	Exhausted at rest; unable to carry out ADL.	Energy to carry out limited activities.	Energy to carry out required and optional activities.
3. Normal nutritional status. Examples of daily meals reflect well-balanced diet; normal weight.	No oral food or fluid intake for two days or more. Inadequate intake to maintain weight.	Dietary intake of poor quantity or quality (less than 800-1200 calories per day) Weight 20% above or below normal.	Calorie intake above 1500 to 3000 calories. Weight within 10% above or below normal.
4. Good (quick) skin turgor, sample intake measurement within required range.	Mucous membranes dry. Skin turgor poor (slow). Fluid intake less than 900 cc/day.	Mucous membranes dry. Skin turgor poor (slow). Fluid intake between 900 to 1900 cc/day.	Mucous membranes moist. Skin turgor good (quick). Fluid intake above 1900 cc per day.
5. Bowels move at intervals, amount and consistency normal to patient. Urinary output is within normal limits for quantity and quality.	No bowel movement for 7 days or more. Watery diarrhea for 2 or more days. 500 cc less/or over 2500. Urinary output 0-400 cc/day.	No bowel movement for 3 to 6 days. Frequent semi-formed stools. Urine output 400-1000 cc/day.	Bowel movements normal (for person) Intervals (1-3 days). Formed stools. Urine output 1000-1500 cc/day.

6. Temperature is within normal range.	Oral temperature 97° or above 100°.	Oral temperature between 97°-98° or 99°-100°.	Oral temperature between 98° and 99°
7. Looks and feels clean; skin, hair, gums.	Strong body odor, cracked dry skin, bleeding lips and gums, dull, brittle hair.	Moderate body odor, dry, intact skin, swollen mucous membranes.	No noticeable body odor, pliable warm skin, intact mucous membranes, glossy hair.
8. Sense of quiet and peace consistent with personal preferences.	Complete withdrawal, agitation, aggression, or hostility.	Verbalizes satisfaction, with some reservations, about environment and regime.	Verbalizes satisfaction with environment relative to activity and regime.
9. Demonstrates ability to move about as needed to maintain preferred life activities.	Completely immobilized and dependent.	Limited mobility by self or with assistance for required activities.	Independent mobility for required and preferred activities.
10. Freedom from pain and discomfort.	Continuous pain or discomfort.	Intermittent pain or discomfort.	Comfortable and pain-free.

SOCIO-PSYCHOLOGICAL

11. Sense of interest and involvement with environment. Responds to environmental stimuli.	No overt response to stimuli; sound, pain, smell, touch.	Overt response to noxious stimuli.	Overt response to all stimuli.
12. Freedom of choice: Power to control one's life as long as it does not interfere with others or place oneself	Unable to make or contribute to decisions which affect one's self.	Offers verbal input to others who make decisions which will affect self.	Able to make decisions and carry them out.

8. Human Needs Assessment Scale* (cont.)

PHYSICAL	POOR 1	MINIMAL 2	GOOD 3
in physical jeopardy.			
13. Sense of achievement in matters of interest; exposure to new things.	Verbalizes no sense of satisfaction or achievement with work, self-development, social life, or personal life. Withdraws from new experiences.	Verbalizes sense of satisfaction or achievement in some areas with some reservations. Participates in new experiences tentatively with strong encouragement.	Verbalizes enthusiasm and satisfaction and can anticipate as well as participate in new experiences.
14. Sense of security and freedom from fear.	Expresses (verbally or non-verbally) fear of people, events & surroundings.	Expresses (verbally or non-verbally) security with environment but fear of people and events.	Expresses (verbally or non-verbally) confidence and security.
15. Knowledge or satisfactory interpretation of the future to enable one to act in one's own best interests.	No knowledge of immediate future.	Can predict short-term future.	Can predict with reasonable confidence both short- and relatively long-term future.
16. Sense of orientation to time, place, person, or situation.	Disoriented to time, place, person, and situation.	Oriented to familiar person.	Completely oriented to time, place, person, and situation.
17. Knowledge of health practices required to maintain satisfactory status.	No participation in self-care.	Participates in self-care with much encouragement.	Verbalizes rationale for and actively participates in self-care.
18. Communication with	No communication with	Communicates with family	Relates to events and people

outside world — family, friends, others, news, TV, etc.	anyone.	and significant others.	in "outside" world as well as family.
19. Sense of recognition, acceptance, respect, and approval re: Status Success Self-esteem	Expresses feelings (verbally or non-verbally) of no status, self rejection, and non-worth.	Expresses feelings of no status or success but can identify some qualities of self-worth.	Expresses (verbally or non-verbally) feeling of self-esteem, and relates incidents of success or status.
20. Sense of desired privacy: Physical Confidential information *ENVIRONMENT*	Communicates feelings of being intruded upon, violated, or embarrassed.	Communicates feelings of being intruded upon, but not feeling violated or embarrassed.	Communicates satisfaction with physical and psycho-social privacy.
21. Can depend on the important things remaining generally the same.	Cannot depend on anything important remaining the same.	Can depend on life, food, and shelter remaining the same in near future.	Can depend on life, food, shelter, and personal relationships remaining stable.
22. Environment is simple, understandable, and controllable.	Completely unable to control environment.	Can express meaning of environment but cannot control it.	Can express meaning of environment and can also control it.
23. Can count on the fact that adjustments can be made as needed and preferred.	Certain that preference will not be considered.	Can bargain for adjustments but cannot be certain of consideration.	Can bargain for adjustment and be assured of consideration.
24. Sense of ability to meet financial requirements to maintain environment.	Certain that others in environment are not safe.	Reasonably certain that most others are safe most of the time.	Certain that others are safe under usual circumstances.

Adapted from Mayers, Norby and Watson: Quality Assurance for Patient Care, Nursing Perspectives, 1977, pp. 119-123. Courtesy of Appleton-Century-Crofts Publishing Co.

9. Nursing History, Extended Care

NAME _____, _____ ADM DATE _____ ATTENDING PHYS _

AGE _____ BIRTHDATE _____ BIRTHPLACE _____ SEX _____

MARITAL STATUS _____ OCCUPATION _____

ACCOMPANIED BY _____ RELATIONSHIP _____ PHONE ___

ADMITTED FROM _____

DIAGNOSIS _____

1. PAIN _____ LOCATION _____ HISTORY OF PAIN _____

2. DOES PATIENT RELATE TO OTHERS? _____

3. EMOTIONAL STATUS

   DEPRESSED☐   WITHDRAWN☐   AGGRESSIVE☐
   ANXIOUS☐   CONFUSED☐

4. IMPAIRED SENSES

   SIGHT☐ HEARING☐ SWALLOWING☐ BALANCE☐

5. SKIN CONDITION

   DEHYDRATED☐   EDEMA☐   DISCOLORATION☐
   BROKEN AREAS☐   PERSONAL HYGIENE☐

6. ALLERGIES _____

7. PROSTHESES _____

   DENTURES   YES☐   NO☐
   GLASSES   YES☐   NO☐
   HEARING AID YES☐   NO☐
   OTHER _____

8. DAILY HABITS:

   A. EATING HABITS: Well☐   Fair☐   Poor☐

      Dislikes _____

      Likes _____
         (as to food, beverages, snacks, etc.)

   B. SLEEPING

      Usual time of arising _____

      Usual time of retiring _____

      Amount of cover at night _____

      Light Room _____ Dark Room _____

      Heavy Sleeper _____ Light Sleeper _____

      How many pillows generally used _____

      Naps _____

   C. BATHING

      Tub _____

Shower _____

Bed Bath _____

Shampoo _____

Shaving: Self _____ Electric _____

D. DRESSING HABITS   *(Specific from head to toe, such as hat, slippers, etc.)*

Helps Self _____

Needs Help _____

9. ELIMINATION HABITS

Does patient take laxatives, regular? What type? _____

10. SOCIAL HABITS

Enjoys group activites _____ Radio _____ TV _____

Prefers to be alone _____

11. HOBBIES

Past occupation _____

Work habits _____

Favorite pastime _____

(Such as reading, handiwork, crafts, etc.)

12. FAMILY

Relationship _____

Who do we call for special needs? _____

What visitors will be coming? _____

_____

13. WE WOULD APPRECIATE ANY OTHER PERTINENT IN-
FORMATION ABOUT YOUR LOVED ONE THAT MAY MAKE
HIS/HER STAY WITH US HAPPIER AND HEALTHIER:

_____

_____

_____

_____

10. Guidelines for Community Assessment

1. GENERAL DESCRIPTION OF COMMUNITY

A. Brief historical background; i.e., major factors which led to present status of community.

B. Environment: Boundaries of community, topography, natural resources, ecology.

C. Physical Structures: Industry, shopping areas, farms, schools, recreation, gathering places, housing, significant conditions; e.g., new developments, condemned housing.

D. Community Services; e.g., transportation, sanitation, fire protection, police, newspaper.

E. Population
   1. Demographic variables including age and sex distribution, income levels, education, religious affiliation, employment, ethnicity, language spoken.
   2. Significant trends, changes in population characteristics.
   3. Power structure: Official government, unofficial leaders.

2. DESCRIPTION OF HEALTH SERVICES AND NEEDS
   A. Health-Care Delivery
      1. Major health-care facilities, agencies, organizations.
      2. Types of nursing roles in health care; e.g., in agencies, innovative roles.
   B. Health Needs and Problems
      1. As indicated by statistics; e.g., births, accidents, morbidity, mortality, incidence, prevalence.
      2. As identified by health-care providers.
      3. As identified by consumers.
   C. Barriers to health care, including factors related to utilization, accessibility, acceptability, quality (also considering cultural variables).

3. RECOMMENDATIONS FOR HEALTH-CARE DELIVERY AND PLANNING (INCLUDING NURSE INVOLVEMENT).
   A. Short-term goals
   B. Long-range planning

Adapted from and courtesy of Kathleen May, R.N., M.S., California State University, Sacramento, Division of Nursing.

Index

A

Algorithms
  cognitive/intellectual system of man, 294
  definition of, 139-141
  demographic systems of environment, 328
  economic system of environment, 316
  examples of, 140, 143, 145, 146, 148, 149, 151, 154, 224
  for assessment, 140, 223, 315
  grand tour questions, 141-155
  interactive/affiliative system of man, 303
  mobile system of environment, 326
  mobile system of man, 309
  physical system of environment, 318
  physiological system of man, 224
  psychological system of man, 287
  sensory/perceptive system of man, 298
  social/cultural system of man, 330
Assessment
  algorithms, 140
  cognitive/intellectual system, 144, 146, 176, 294-297
  definition, 4
  economic system, 316-317
  examples of, 64-69, 125-130, 131, 136, 155-158
  guides, 60-63
  interactive/affiliative system, 147, 149, 150, 155-158, 177, 182-187, 302-308
  mobile system, 150-152, 163, 166-169, 177, 188-189, 309-312, 326-327
  physical system, 318-325
  physiological system, 142-143, 176, 225-286
  process of, 29
  psychological system, 142, 144-145, 176, 288-293
  sensory/perceptive system, 147-148, 177, 190-192, 299-302
  social/cultural system, 153, 155-156, 330-332
  theories for, 16-18
  theory-based, 58, 59
  theory-based guides, 204, 208

G

Grand tour questions, 33, 141-155, 176-181

H

Health
definition of, 34
standards of cognitive/intellectual, 295-297
standards of demographic, 329
standards of economic, 317
standards of interactive/affiliative, 60-69, 125-130, 131-136, 182-187, 302-308
standards of mobile, 188, 310-312, 372
standards of physical, 319-325
standards of physiological, 225-286
standards of psychological, 288-293
standards of sensory/perceptive, 190
standards of social/cultural, 331-332
Hypotheses, 21

I

Inference
definition of, 28
examples of, 64-69
Inspecting, 28
Interactive/affiliative system of man
algorithm for assessment of, 149
assessment case study, 147, 150, 155-158
assessment guide for, 60-63, 182-187
health standards, 60-69, 125-130, 131-136
theories of, 15, 60-63

J

Judgments, 21

M

N

O

P

Physical system of environment
  algorithm for assessment, 318
  health standards, 319-325
Physiological system of man
  algorithm for assessment of, 143-224
  assessment case study, 142
  health standards, 225-286
Policy formulation
  for the client, 208, 213, 216-217
  for the employee, 215-216
  for evaluation, 216, 218-219
  for the provider, 214-215, 217-218
Problem oriented documentation
  description of, 77-79
  examples of, 80-83, 105-109, 113-115, 159-163
Psychological system of man
  algorithm for assessment of, 145
  assessment case study, 142, 144
  health standards, 288-293

Q

Questioning
  description of, 27, 28
  grand tour, 33, 176-181

R

Referrals, 91, 92
Research
  deductive, 2, 3
  inductive, 2, 3

S

Sensory/perceptive system of man
  algorithm for assessment of, 148
  assessment case study, 147

T